<u>Introduction – Who?</u>

A book designed for all first time mums
all the information I gathered when I was pregnant.

I am a first time mum, having given birth in February 2014 to a beautiful little girl Sumaya. Yes we do all say our children are beautiful.

I had a fairly easy pregnancy but this didn't stop me from gathering a lot of information about what to expect since I was expecting.

I'm definitely one of those women that like to know everything. I like to go to appointments prepared. I want to know what's coming up so that anything the doctor or nurse has to say is simply a confirmation of what I already knew. As a result throughout my pregnancy and into the first few months of motherhood I've done a whole load of research. From morning sickness in trimester one, to pain relief in labour, I've got a little knowledge about a lot of things baby related.

I'm by no means a doctor nor do I claim to be a professional but what I do know is I've been where you are and I've shared in at least some of your experiences, both past and yet to come.

I'd like to note, I will mention products and websites throughout this book but it's not an advertising campaign. You are free to choose whichever product you feel suits you and your baby best. I can only speak from experience and pass on what I have learnt in the short time I have been a mother.

I can guarantee that you will take at least something out of this book, whether it be information on what you're currently going through or information on what's likely to come up over the next few months.

I may have only been a mum for a short period of time but I do feel confident in my new found role. I put this down to the amount of research I did on what to expect and how to manage. I may not always make the best decisions but I do make very well informed ones.

This is unlike any other pregnancy book in that I am simply passing on what I know. I want all you new and not so new mums to feel informed, to feel confident and to feel prepared.

<u>Most importantly though I wish all my Yummy Mummy's to be a happy and healthy 9 months</u>

0 - 3 Months – First Trimester

So if you're reading this, you've most likely had a positive pregnancy test.

Whether at home or in the doctor's surgery you've seen those precious two lines, cross or 'Pregnant' appear on a test. For many the reaction can be a mix of Joy, Fear, Excitement, and Confusion. It may be all or none of the above. For the most part it's all pretty normal.

For the first two weeks of pregnancy though, you weren't actually pregnant. They count pregnancy from the date of your last period, and for many you wouldn't have ovulated for approximately 14 days. There is some science behind it, but for the most part it's pretty irrelevant other than to know that's why when they give you your due date they call it an EDD – Expected Due Date.

It's wise if you've only had a home test to book an appointment with your GP to both confirm the pregnancy and arrange a referral to the midwife for your booking appointment

False positives are very rare though so it is very likely the GP will simply confirm you really are pregnant.

Changes to your body

As with anything relating to an individual, pregnancy can affect women in different ways. What may be your experience this trimester may be completely different to another woman's. You may be full of energy and glowing or feeling miserable and drained.

Bleeding in pregnancy

About a ¼ of women bleed at some point during the first trimester. By bleed I don't mean anything close to a period but more like light spotting. This, specifically in the first few weeks may be what's called implantation bleeding. Implantation bleeding is where the fertilised embryo implants itself in your uterus. However, any significant bleeding especially alongside pains in your uterus or abdomen needs medical assistance - usually a GP can advise or failing that a call to NHS Direct.

Bleeding unfortunately can be a sign of either a miscarriage or an ectopic pregnancy

Miscarriages are classed as a pregnancy loss occurring on or before the 20th week of pregnancy. Approximately 20% of all pregnancies end in a miscarriage. A miscarriage can occur for a number of different reasons, although it is not always possible to tell. It may be something genetic, an infection, and an abnormality that occurred or none of the above. Bleeding is often the most common symptom of a miscarriage. This can be light and brown or heavy and bright red.

Approximately 50% of women that seek medical assistance for bleeding in pregnancy will miscarry

A suspected miscarriage can be confirmed through an ultrasound exam (a scan), an internal exam – to see if the cervix is open or tests on your HCG levels (HCG levels are what indicate pregnancy on pregnancy tests).

If confirmed you may be offered treatment.

The treatment of a miscarriage is as follows:

- No treatment at all – in most cases the embryo will pass naturally within 6 weeks
- Medical management using tablets to encourage completion of the natural process
- Surgical treatment – i.e. an operation to remove the contents of the uterus.

An Ectopic pregnancy is somewhat different though and can be life threatening. It's where the embryo plants itself outside of the womb. In most cases it can be found in one of the fallopian tubes. One of the main causes of an ectopic pregnancy is PID (Pelvic Inflammatory Disease) an infection of the female reproductive system. PID is caused by bacteria most commonly the STD Chlamydia.

Unfortunately ectopic pregnancies are not always detected. They may not be realised until an early scan shows a problem, or the situation becomes life threatening. If there are symptoms though, one of the signs can be abnormal vaginal bleeding and abdominal pain. If present, in most cases the abdominal pain is one sided.

If an ectopic pregnancy is suspected, an ultrasound will be performed to see if the ectopic can be located. As this happens very early on in a pregnancy it will often be a vaginal ultrasound. A small probe is inserted to take an image of your womb and the surrounding areas. Blood tests may also be used to measure your HCG levels. Ectopic pregnancies and miscarriages tend to have below average HCG levels.

If confirmed it is important to understand the baby cannot be saved.

It is very important the pregnancy be terminated as soon as possible. If detected early enough the ectopic pregnancy can be treated with an injection of methotrexate. In ½ of all cases though your body will realise something isn't right and the egg dies naturally. However, if the egg continues to grow it will need to be treated. If left untreated it can cause life threatening internal bleeding. This can occur when the fertilised egg ruptures the fallopian tube.

Signs of a ruptured fallopian tube:

- Pain in the tip of your shoulder
- Dizziness or fainting
- Sudden, sharp pain
- Diarrhoea

A ruptured fallopian tube will require surgery to remove part if not all of your fallopian tube. It is classed as a medical emergency and an ambulance should be called.

It is now very uncommon for an ectopic pregnancy to result in death but approximately 1 in 90 pregnancies do end up being ectopic in the UK.

Breasts, Boobies, Bosoms

For many, breast tenderness was their first sign of pregnancy. Breasts will often feel tender and swollen. Even at this stage your milk ducts are growing in preparation for all the breastfeeding you'll be doing later. For me they were extremely sensitive, especially the nipple area. I chose to pack away my fancy underwire bras opting for the more comfortable sports bra.

By the end of the first trimester your nipple area might become dark especially if you have darker hair or are of a darker complexion. Your nipples may also be slightly larger and have more pronounced little bumps.

The only thing I can suggest to reduce soreness is to make sure you wear a supportive bra. Cotton bras are more comfortable and breathable. Your breasts will continue to change shape so underwires are not recommended.

If it gets really bad you may need to invest in a pregnancy sleep bra – which you should be able to buy in the likes of Mothercare and Babies 'r' us.

It's probably not a good idea to spend mass amounts of money on them though. As your belly grows your breasts will also – probably by about 2 sizes. By the time you give birth you'll need nursing bras anyway, especially if you're considering breastfeeding.

Sleep – well lack of it anyway

Even from the first trimester you'll begin to feel tired during the day. You'll find yourself yawning at work and in desperate need of a nap. I found myself clockwatching by 3pm, day dreaming about the comfortable bed I had waiting at home for me. I've never been one to fall asleep on public transport but in the first few month of pregnancy, I could fall asleep standing.

You'd think with this tiredness you'd get a great night's sleep. In actual fact you might even begin to have trouble sleeping at night, blame it on those hormones – progesterone in this case.

As well as the hormone, your new painful breasts might make it difficult to get comfortable. Things will only get more uncomfortable so it's probably best to try start sleeping on your left side from now. Sleeping on your left side is best for your baby's oxygen levels, it helps with the flow of blood and nutrients from you to your baby.

Your uterus is also growing at speed to accommodate your growing baby which adds extra pressure to your bladder. This means plenty of trips to the bathroom. If at work it's probably the hardest pregnancy sign to hide. To stop this interrupting your sleep try not to drink too much in the afternoon and into the evening.

For a more comfortable sleep you also might want to invest in a pregnancy sleep pillow. If you're going to buy it from now you might want one with washable covers. They are multi-functional and can later be used as a nursing pillow.

No matter what happens though just try to remember your body is going through a lot of changes and is working really hard. Listen to your body, when you're tired, rest.

Pregnancy and your skin

Unfortunately that widely celebrated pregnancy glow doesn't come around until the second trimester. Up until then pregnancy may play havoc on your skin.

Got to love those hormones because right with them comes acne. It's down to your skin producing more oil which can cause you to revisit those adolescent years you'd rather forget. Not to worry though, the pimples and bumps should settle down over time.

In the meantime try to avoid scrubbing or over washing your skin. It's also the perfect opportunity to try out an oil free natural moisturiser.

Nausea – The dreaded morning sickness

For me, morning sickness was the worst pregnancy symptom. What made it worse was that it wasn't and isn't only in the morning. Okay, so in fairness to its name, the morning was the worst part of the day for me. As soon as I tried to get out of bed it would be a mad dash to the toilets to vomit. Worse than the actual vomiting was the constant and persistent nausea.

Morning Sickness affects at least 75% of mums to be. If your one of the lucky few to have escaped unscathed count yourself lucky. There are some tips I compiled through my research that helped me get through the first few months.

- Salt crackers by your bed – like a box of RITZ - these should be eaten while in bed, 20 mins or so before you have to get up
- Sitting up in bed before you get out for a few minutes
- Ginger tea or ginger cubes from a health food store like Holland and Barrett's
- Sea sick band – bought from most chemists – make sure you put it on correctly. They work by hitting pressure points.
- Eating small meals often rather than 3 main meals
- Drinking lemonade or sucking on lemon sweets
- Rest – tiredness can make morning sickness worse
- Acupuncture – I personally don't have an experience but I have heard great things about its success.

If it gets really bad and nothing seems to be working you may need your GP to prescribe anti-sickness medicine called an antiemetic.

It's time to contact your GP if you haven't been able to keep any food or drink down in 24 hours.

Round Ligament Pain

This was a really painful part of the first trimester for me. When it first began I thought I was having an ectopic pregnancy and rushed to the EPAU – Early pregnancy Assessment Unit for an emergency transvaginal scan. A probe was inserted and my tubes checked for an ectopic. In actual fact the embryo had planted itself in my womb and Sumaya was well on her way to developing.

I was left with a new question then, what the hell was causing all the pain? It was like nothing I'd ever experienced before. I was told it was 'normal' and growing pains like I was an adolescent having a growth spurt.

As mentioned in my introduction, I like to know as much as I can about anything that concerns me so telling me 'it's normal' is simply not cutting it. I headed straight from the EPAU to the library to research.

I realised I was experiencing round ligament pain. As my uterus was growing it was causing the short jabbing pains whenever I changed positions. Literally I was in pain when I got out of bed, got in the shower, got out the shower, coughed, got in and out of a chair. Literally I was in pain whenever I moved. The pain was around the groin and hip area and sometimes felt like muscle pain. I felt like I had done a 3 hour Zumbathon where I'd been shaking my bom bom a little too hard.

It was confirmed that round ligament pain is very common but shouldn't be confused with severe pain or cramping.

The only thing that can help with this pain is bringing your knees up to your belly when possible. You will find ways around the pain and to be honest knowing it was normal kind of made it easier to deal with because it wasn't affecting the baby.

Foods in pregnancy

There are a number of foods that should be avoided in pregnancy. I know right? First you can't keep much down and then there's a limit to what you're actually allowed to eat.

- Some Cheeses: Brie, Camembert as they may contain listeria. You don't want any cheese made with unpasteurised milk.
- Pate: all types including vegetarian as they may contain listeria
- Raw or undercooked eggs: this includes both the white and yolk parts. Be particularly mindful of homemade mayonnaise and raw eggs in mousse.
- Raw or undercooked meat: There should be no remaining pink or bloody meat. This includes cured meats such as Parma Ham.
- Fish: You are allowed one portion of oily fish a week and 4 cans of Tuna. Oily fish can be high in pollutants and Tuna can contain levels of mercury which can be damaging to baby. Fish such as shark, swordfish and marlin should be avoided. Also – NO SUSHI or undercooked fish at all.
- Caffeine: Caffeine should be limited. If possible you may want to cut it out altogether – I know it will be hard following the crazy fatigue.
- Alcohol: There is some confusion about what's safe in pregnancy and what's not, so probably best to cut it out altogether or limit it to one or 2 units a week

So what exactly is listeria and what affects can it have on both you and your unborn child?

Listeria is a type of bacteria that contaminates vegetables from the soil. Animals can also be carriers although in both cases the listeria is killed through the cooking process. Listeriosis (the illness caused by the Listeria) is rare but with pregnancy lowering your defences pregnant women are more susceptible. Symptoms of Listeriosis include headaches, fever, nausea and vomiting although a blood test will be needed to confirm any infection.

If found to have Listeriosis you are at an increased risk of miscarriage, premature delivery and neonatal death. Listeriosis is easily treatable with antibiotics and in most cases this will prevent infection to the baby.

Enough of the don'ts, here's a few **superfoods** to consume when pregnant.

- Broccoli: Super vegetable – half your daily recommendation of Vitamin C and Potassium. Great for the digestive system – Take that Pregnancy Constipation
- Strawberries – A great pregnancy snack, high in iron – will help fight pregnancy fatigue
- Salmon – Great for your little one's brain and vision development
- Cabbage – Great for vitamins and minerals including folic acid. Cabbage leaves chilled can be placed in your bra to soothe breasts after nursing.
- Sweet Potatoes – An excellent source of folic acid – try baking like a jacket potato
- Almonds – Packed full of unsaturated fats critical for your little ones brain

Booking Appointment

The booking appointment is normally the first time you will meet with the midwife normally at around 8 weeks although it can be as late as 10th. This is mainly due to the fact that the chance of miscarriage is quite high up to this point.

The booking appointment can be quite a lengthy appointment and pretty intrusive. It's basically a really long computerised form filled in by the midwife. You'll be asked your last period date so they can work out and document your EDD. Probably best to already know this as it does carry you through for the next 9 months. You are asked about your previous sexual history in terms of any previous pregnancies. These include miscarriages, abortions, ectopic pregnancies, still and live births. It's important to be as open as possible about these as it allows the midwife to advise you about any additional antenatal care you might need.

In most areas there will be a few different choices on where you intend on having your baby. Any complications may limit your choice though for the safety of you and your baby. It's therefore important to be as open as possible with your midwife even if previous pregnancies are difficult to talk about. The different options available in the UK to give birth are covered in the 6-9 months section of this book.

Next there is a whole section on family history. Mainly covering immediate family i.e. parents, grandparents, siblings (on both sides) you'll be asked about any diabetes, high blood pressure, heart disease and even mental health problems in the family.

The rest isn't as intrusive to be honest.
There's a section covering your job – not because they want to offer career advice or anything. It's in case you have a job that might have additional risks that could affect your pregnancy i.e. if it involves strenuous work or involving physically demanding tasks that might prove difficult towards the end of the pregnancy.

Please note though – it's your employer's responsibility once informed of your pregnancy to find you alternative work at the same rate of pay

You'll also be asked about your alcohol intake and whether you smoke. Smoking in pregnancy can have adverse effects on your baby. It can lead to your baby having a lower birth weight which in turn increases the risk of your baby being stillborn or disabled. It can also cause miscarriage or premature labour. Your midwife can offer you information and advice on quitting and even refer you to external departments trained in assisting women to quit. To show the importance of this issue there is now a free helpline specifically for smoking in pregnancy run by the NHS – 0800 169 9169.

If you haven't started, you will need to begin taking folic acid. You will be asked about this, and given information on its benefits.

Folic Acid ideally should be taken before you fall pregnant but if not, you need to take it as soon as you find out. You need approximately 400mcgs of folic acid to help protect your unborn baby from developing birth defects. Mainly it helps prevents against Spina Bifida which is also known as split spine.

Spina Bifida is basically a fault in the development of the spine and can result in a wide range of symptoms from reading problems, to muscle weakness and paralysis as well as bladder and bowel incontinence. The exact cause of Spina Bifida isn't known but a lack of folic acid in the first month of pregnancy has been found to increase the risk.
As well as taking a supplement you can also get folic acid from folate rich foods such as: orange juice, broccoli, brussel sprouts and baked potatoes.

You are given a lot of information in this first appointment. As well as supplement and vitamin advice you will be advised on exercise in pregnancy, any antenatal classes available and the importance of healthy eating.

Once the form has been filled in this may be printed off and stored in your folder. Each hospital seems to have a different coloured folder for their pregnant women. This folder will store all your information regarding your pregnancy from your scan information and results to notes written at your antenatal appointments.

They tend to have a timeline page detailing the frequency of your antenatal appointments and what to expect at each visit. For the most part the below is followed for a first time mum. These will not always be with a midwife and may increase in frequency depending on any complications.

10 Weeks – Booking Appointment
12 Weeks – Dating Scan
16 Weeks – Discuss results of screening tests
20 Weeks – Anomaly Scan
25 Weeks
28 Weeks – Measure the bump with a tape measure and offer more screening tests
31 Weeks – Discuss results of screening tests
34 Weeks – Information on preparing for labour
36 Weeks – Information on caring for yourself and baby after labour
38 Weeks – Information on what happens if pregnancy goes past 41 weeks
40 Weeks
41 Weeks (if you still haven't given birth) – Offer of membrane sweep and discuss options of induction
In the folder there will also be pages of sticky labels. These will have your details on them including name, date of birth and NHS number. These are used to send off any blood and urine tests.

At the booking appointment you will get blood taken so if you're afraid of needles or anything like that it might be worth taking someone with you. You will be have your blood group tested, your iron levels checked, measles immunisation confirmed and rhesus status noted.

Rhesus status can be either positive or negative. If your RhD negative carrying an RhD positive baby you will need anti-D injections into your upper arm to prevent your baby's blood cells being attacked. These are very important and will be offered at 28 and 34 weeks pregnant. Most people are RhD positive but if you are not your midwife will be able to provide you with more information.

You may also have your blood screened for HIV, syphilis and Hepatitis B although you can choose to opt out of these if you wish.

As well as blood tests your urine will be tested for protein. This is something you will quickly become accustomed to as it is done at nearly all future appointments. Protein found in the urine can be an indication of dehydration; a urine infection; kidney disorder, high blood pressure diabetes and later on in the pregnancy pre eclampsia. Don't be too concerned though, as sometimes a small reading of protein may simply be a contaminated sample.

Your blood pressure is another check done at most antenatal appointments. High blood pressure is also an indication of pre eclampsia or an indication of something else needing to be investigated. Your blood pressure will be noted at each appointment in your folder.
The only other check really at this stage will be your BMI, so your height and weight. This will be to ensure you have as healthy a pregnancy as possible. If its high (over 30) you will need to ensure your diet is healthy as a high BMI can lead to gestational diabetes. Too low (under 18) increases the risk of a baby being born with a low birth weight which again carries its own complications.

You may also be given information on signs you should never ignore during this trimester such as vaginal bleeding, abdominal pain etc.

Make sure you get your maternity exemption certificate stamped at this appointment. It is a form sent away that will enable you to get free prescriptions and dental care both during your pregnancy and until your baby is one year old.

Before you leave you will also be given information on your dating scan. This may be arranged via your midwife but in most cases you will either receive a letter or have a number to call to arrange.

Dating Scan

Providing the pregnancy hasn't had any complications you will be offered your first scan between 10 and 13 weeks. This is known as a dating scan.

Although an exciting time as it's often the first opportunity to see your baby on screen, the scan is used to establish your due date.

The sonographer will put gel on your tummy and move a hand held device over your abdomen. I remember being shocked at how low the device seemed to be and was grateful to be wearing a top and trousers rather than a dress.

The sonographer may point out the parts of your baby on a screen indicating which parts of the body are where.

The scan is also used to measure your baby's length (at this stage, its head to bottom called Crown Rump Length or CRL). You will also see how many babies you are carrying and confirm the heartbeat.

The heartbeat can be seen as a flicking light, it's initially quite strange but very reassuring as you can actually see it beating away.

If you want to have a picture printed out as a keepsake you will have to ask for this before the scan begins. You may also need to pay for this service and most hospitals don't tend to have card machines so you'll need to have some cash handy.

During the dating scan you may be offered the combined test where a measurement is taken of the fluid at the back of the baby's neck. If you are not offered it, you may want to mention it. It may be that your midwife has already indicated that it should be done on the scan paper.

The combined test is known as the nuchal translucency scan and is an assessment of your baby's risk of Down's syndrome. For this to be offered you will have to be between 11 and 13 weeks + 6 Pregnant (13 weeks + 6 literally means 13 weeks + 6 days, so 1 day under 14 weeks). As well as the measurement taken you may also need a blood test done, this is done for increased accuracy and shouldn't be a cause for concern.

In the unlikely event that the sonographer believes there is a higher risk for Down's syndrome or any other chromosomal abnormalities you will be offered additional tests such as CVS (Chorionic Villus Sampling).

CVS can confirm any chromosomal abnormalities or suspected cases of Down's syndrome. It should be noted though that the majority of referrals result in the case being negative.

CVS is basically a thin needle inserted (under local anaesthetic) inserted into your uterus to take some cells from the placenta. These are then taken away and analysed for the chromosomal makeup (including sex) of your baby. There are both risks and advantages of this procedure all of which will be discussed in detail with you before you are expected to make a decision on whether to have the procedure performed or not.

The First Trimester summed up

In short the first 3 months of pregnancy can be the most difficult. Your body is going through a lot of changes. Hormones coupled with a lack of sleep and morning sickness can lead to an emotional rollercoaster. One minute you may be feeling excited and happy and the next angry or tearful. Rest assured it will get easier and you will adapt. If you are concerned though please do reach out to your midwife or GP. I'm pretty sure there's not much they haven't heard before and they are there to help. It may also help to join an online group of other pregnant woman. I spent many weeks and months and even now trailing through forums of other pregnant mums reading their rants and complaints. It can really help you to not feel alone and to feel that there are other people going through what you are. I personally recommend the below although there are many out there:

http://community.babycentre.co.uk/
http://www.netmums.com/coffeehouse/pregnancy-64/
http://www.mumsnet.com/Talk/pregnancy

3 - 6 Months – Second Trimester

You've made it! The Second Trimester for me was my favourite. It was the time to enjoy the pregnancy before the worry of labour and parenthood.

Although a miscarriage is a loss of the foetus before the 20th week of pregnancy, the chance of miscarriage in the second trimester (known as a late miscarriage) is less than 10%. Knowing this gave me a sense of relief. I could relax slightly and begin to enjoy the pregnancy.

If I could have implemented two tips into my life in the 2nd trimester they would have been keeping up with my water intake and exercising regularly. Exercise is looked at later but in terms of the water intake this should be at a minimum 1.5L a day. Water prevents urine infections and constipation. It helps the baby get the necessary nutrients and stops you retaining water. If you're already getting swollen chances are you may be dehydrated.

The majority of women tend to enjoy the second trimester due to the nausea and tiredness fading. Your bump might not be to big either yet so moving around should still be relatively easy.

The second trimester in all is an exciting time, you'll have another scan, (maybe even find out the sex). You'll also reach your midway point – Yayy!! By the end of the second trimester you will definitely have a bump of some kind to have to dress for – more shopping!! You're also very likely to feel your baby move at some point.

Spreading the news

Telling friends and family

You've gotten past the initial danger zone so if you haven't already now might be the time to let people know. You could always send around a broadcast on the likes of WhatsApp or SMS text message. On the other hand here is a list of fun ways I've found for people letting their friends and family know.

- A photo of you reading a book (maybe even this one, hey free publicity, support a first time mum)
- A photo of you shopping for little shoes or other pregnancy related item such as breast pads
- One of those coloured cakes, with the colour pink or blue once you cut into it – if you choose to find out the sex at 20 weeks
- With a baby bump photo – one for the collection
- Do a Beyoncé cover and post a video on you tube – maybe without the so called collapsing baby bump though
- A broadcast begging for your latest crazy craving – pickles and ice cream anyone?
- Announce with invitations to the baby shower

Informing your work

You have to tell your work about your pregnancy by the 15th week before your expected due date. Most people will have told their employer before then due to antenatal appointments etc.

The law states you are allowed to take off time for antenatal appointments without losing any pay. This includes any time to travel to the clinic or surgery. Your employer will need what is called a MATB1 Certificate signed or stamped by your GP or midwife

You should get this around the 20th week of pregnancy but if not you can ask your midwife to provide one. The MATB1 is basically a piece of paper confirming your pregnancy and due date.

Depending on how long you've worked for your employer you may be entitled to SMP (Statutory maternity pay). Your HR department should be able to provide the details of this.

If you do not qualify for SMP due to how long you've worked there you may be able to claim maternity allowance. Details for this should be available from your local job centre or citizens advice bureau.

Changes to your body

Baby Bump

During the second trimester your baby is going to grow rapidly. At the end of this book is a chart showing the average length and weight of your baby at each week. Between 14 and 26 weeks your baby goes from 8cm to 35 and 43g to 760. This rapid growth means your stomach is also going to grow too (although not necessarily at the same speed).

With this growing bump you may begin to notice stretch marks appearing on your thighs, stomach and breasts. I don't know of any creams or lotions that actually work 100% but I do recommend Bio Oil and Cocoa butter. They will eventually fade overtime after delivery and become less noticeable. I've fully accepted they will never be invisible but for me I view them as a mark of motherhood, something to be proud of.

Even with an ever growing body be careful not to overeat, you actually only need 300-500 calories extra per day in the second trimester and should be gaining on average ½ - 1 pound a week.

Exercise in pregnancy

Weight gain can best be controlled if you exercise throughout pregnancy. If you've not been someone to exercise regularly before pregnancy don't go trying to start an intensive exercise program but some can still be introduced. Before you start any exercise program you should consult your GP.

I wish I had been in a better physical state before I fell pregnant and had realised the benefits of exercise during but all in hindsight I suppose.

Swimming is the most recommended form of exercise during pregnancy. Not only is this a safe way to exercise but the water will support your weight especially as your bump gets bigger. It will also help to keep your ligaments stretched and as nimble as possible. Another highly recommended exercise is Yoga. It not only helps with aches and pains but will help to keep your mind relaxed.

The most important rule when exercising though is to stay hydrated and not over exert yourself. If you can hold a conversation comfortably while exercising you should be fine. If you do decide to attend a fitness class of some kind, be sure to inform the teacher (properly qualified of course) that you are pregnant.

There are some rules when exercising in pregnancy though:

- Don't lie flat on your back after 16 weeks
- No contact sports where there is a risk of being hit – i.e. boxing, squash etc.
- No exercises that have a risk of falling – horse riding, ice skating, etc.

Baby movements

My absolute favourite part of pregnancy was feeling Sumaya moving about. This begins with flutter type movements, a bit like butterflies in your tummy. It may initially be put down to gas but by the end of your pregnancy there will be no denying the power kicks and punches of your little one.

Most women will feel some type of movement from their baby by the end of the second trimester. There are a number of different factors that can affect how soon you will notice these movements but as with everything it's different for all women. If it's your first pregnancy you are likely to feel the baby move later than someone who has already had a baby. This may be because the second or third time mum may know what to look out for. Body shape can also play a role in how quickly you'll notice baby movement.

Placenta position was a factor for me, Sumaya would often kick into the placenta which was acting as a cushion between her and me.

One thing I wish I had known is that you will soon know what's normal for your baby. You can't really compare the amount of movement you have versus someone else. I spent many hours wasting time on forums trying to figure out if what I was experiencing was normal for my week of pregnancy.

At the beginning you may expect continuous movement. Try to remember how small the baby still is and therefore just because you can't feel movement doesn't mean your little one isn't moving around. If you are concerned at all though your midwife can advise and reassure you.

As the months progress the movements are a lot more noticeable. Kicks really feel like kicks, elbow jabs in the ribs and little wriggles, they are all normal. You may even find yourself thinking 'Ouch' if they hit a tender spot. By the 6th month I was adamant that she had bruised me at least once from the inside.

By the end of the second trimester your baby is likely to have its routine, particularly if you follow a similar routine every day.

What's crazy though is the baby is likely to be more active at night as you are resting preparing to sleep. With you up and down walking around throughout the day your body motions rock your baby to sleep. Even if your baby is awake you may not notice it during the day if you're busy.

I'd found myself at my desk at work thinking, 'Ohh when did she last move'. I'd begin panicking before realising she was moving and I just hadn't noticed because I was caught up on whatever the task may have been.

I did pick up a few tricks along the way though to push Maymay to move when she was being particularly stubborn.

- Eat a snack – the increase in blood sugar should cause the baby to start moving around
- Orange Juice – don't know what it was about the orange juice but this always worked
- Lay down on your left side (if at home of course)
- Relax – it may be you just needed to pay attention and tune into your body

Midwife Appointments

Although it may vary slightly you will have a few midwife/GP appointments during this trimester. The second trimester is counted as sometime after the 12th week (there is some disagreement and it is anytime during the 12, 13, and 14th week) and the 27th week.
There will be a number of antenatal appointments for you to attend either at home or at a clinic. The midwife and GP (if you end up seeing one) will have a quick look at your scan results from your dating scan.

This isn't the actual image as this may not be present depending on whether you purchased one or not. It is a report of measurements and notes from the sonographer. If you haven't already received your results from the NT measurement they will be able to bring this up on the computer – got to love modern technology. The result is given in a fraction, for example Sumaya's was 1/150,000.

This basically meant she had a 1 in 150,000 chance of having Down's syndrome. As a result no further tests were offered.

You will be asked very similar if not exactly the same questions at each visit:

1. How are you feeling? – this is normally about your general well being
2. Are you still feeling sick or suffering from morning sickness?
3. Have you felt the baby move yet? – If they already know the answer to this they may ask you if the baby is moving normally.

Your urine will also be checked for protein. From what I understood this is mainly to check for signs of a urine infection, preeclampsia or gestational diabetes all of which may show protein in your urine. An important note (one I wish I had known!) it is normal to have a small amount of protein in your urine on occasion and shouldn't be a cause for concern.

Protein in the urine can also be linked to dehydration or a contaminated sample. If you continued to have protein though you may have gestational diabetes. This may be checked for anyone at the end of the second trimester by way of blood test.

As well as this your blood pressure will also be checked and noted in your folder. Blood pressure as well as protein in your urine can be a sign of preeclampsia.

Your weight is also recorded as part of the standard antenatal checks. For me this was particularly important. I had a high BMI prior to getting pregnant (33 for all those that are interested) as a result it was important I watch my calorie intake as being obese can increase your chances of getting preeclampsia or gestational diabetes. If you don't have any issues regarding your weight it isn't always necessary to know how much weight you are putting on – especially if you have a fairly balanced diet anyway. The midwife can log your information in the folder and raise it as an issue if they are concerned.

As well as my weight checked at ever appointment I had what is called a RBS. This stands for a random blood sample. It was used to monitor my blood sugar levels and make sure I hadn't developed gestational diabetes. My urine was also more thoroughly scrutinised with any minimal readings being sent away for further analysis. Luckily neither developed but with these as potential illnesses I made sure I knew all the facts.

Preeclampsia

Before I go into what Preeclampsia is, please note only 5% of pregnancies are affected.

It also tends to develop around the 20th week of pregnancy with most cases being seen at around 37 weeks. Some cases even develop during labour or shortly after delivery.

Preeclampsia causes the blood vessels to constrict reducing blood flow to your vital organs including your brain. This therefore means less blood flow to your uterus and therefore your baby. This can result in little growth for the baby and maybe even premature labour.

With the blood vessels in your kidneys leaking protein in your bloodstream spill into your urine, hence the urine tests at your antenatal appointments. The most common symptom is high blood pressure though so this is also tested at your appointments.

Unfortunately preeclampsia can sometimes be quite unpredictable. It may develop slowly or rapidly with mild or severe life threating symptoms. It all depends on the individual to be honest. There are some warning signs though.

Such warning signs include:

- Sudden swelling or puffiness in face and eyes, face, feet
- Rapid weight gain (more than 5lbs a week)
- Severe headache/migraine that won't go away
- Blurred vision or seeing spots
- Upper abdominal pain and tenderness (intense)
- Nausea and vomiting

It may also be an idea to share these with your support network. I was constantly asking my other half if my face or hands were extremely swollen.

Treatment of preeclampsia depends on the severity of the condition and the number of weeks pregnant you are. Most important will be the health of both you and your baby. Whatever advice is given by the health professionals I advise you to make sure you are given all the facts both best and worst outcomes.

Gestational Diabetes

This is one of the most common pregnancy complications affecting up to 10% of women.

Diabetes is about the amount of sugar in your blood. The glucose in the food you eat acts as a fuel to run your body. The glucose is changed into fuel using insulin. Gestational diabetes occurs because your cells are less responsive to the insulin. This is as a result of hormones but for most women isn't too much of a problem. The pancreas just produces more insulin to balance it out. However if your pancreas isn't able to keep up with the demand gestational diabetes occurs because now you have too much glucose in your system unconverted.

Importantly once you give birth you should go back to normal as your body returns to normal. After birth, nursing your baby (breastfeeding) has been found to help prevent childhood obesity and have a positive effect on glucose management.

You're at higher risk if your obese (BMI over 30, like I was), had gestational diabetes in a previous pregnancy, have a family history of diabetes. A study was also done that found non-white women are at a higher risk.

Gestational diabetes is easily managed with diet and sugar control.

A well balanced diet with exercise can really help in the management of gestational diabetes.

If poorly managed your baby may put on extra weight. In severe cases the baby may be too large to enter the birth canal. This may in result in delivery by caesarean.

Anomaly Scale

Between 18 – 20 weeks you will be offered an anomaly screen. This was my favourite of the two standard scans. The main purpose of the scan is to check on the development of your baby

It can be a time of mixed emotions, both fear and excitement. I remember initially finding the whole situation quite daunting. I hadn't seen her in 2 months but I'd begun to feel her move. Now I was going to see her again and how she had changed!
You could see so much more at this scan. Arms, legs, a head with features. It's a pretty beautiful experience. I remember being shocked at the detail. I could see her rib cage, and her moving around. It was both beautiful but surreal.

It was like the pregnancy actually was real and it dawned on me that I was going to be a mum, sooner than I thought.

Don't be worried if your sonographer is quiet, they have to spend a little time making sure everything is okay. Again you will have the option to request images be printed. The report will be placed into your folder with their findings.

Importantly though (for you more so than the sonographer) you may be given the option of finding out the gender of your baby. I know in some hospitals its policy not to tell you as a result of gender selection but your midwife should have informed you about this before your scan.

Whether you find out the gender or not, through choice or policy the scan is another opportunity to check on the development and wellbeing of your unborn child.

The sonographer will be looking at the baby's heart, their face, their spine, kidneys, stomach and abdomen. Measurements will also be taken to ensure they are in line with the number of weeks you were thought to be from the dating scan.

The measurements include head circumference, abdominal circumference and thigh bone length.

Away from the actual baby the sonographer will also note how the placenta is lying. If it's lying low you will have another scan in the third trimester to check its position. This will be to make sure it's moved away from your cervix. If it's lying low it's called Placenta Praevia.

Placenta Praevia

There can be partial placenta praevia which doesn't tend to lead to any complications. If the placenta is covering your cervix at the third trimester scan this may be more complicated.

There is a risk of bleeding that can lead to premature labour and in worst case scenarios a haemorrhage. This is very rare though and with the advances in medicine now quickly treated.

If you are found to have placenta praevia you will be advised to not have sexual intercourse and providing you're not bleeding to stay at home and rest. You may be offered a planned caesarean.

This will be done by a senior doctor and the upmost will be done to ensure the wellbeing of you and the baby.

I know it's easy to worry but there isn't anything you can do to prevent where the placenta is lying. All you can do is be in the best health you can be with the condition. Eat foods high in iron to prevent your iron levels falling or you becoming anaemic. Other than that drink loads of water and rest.

There is always a chance that the placenta will move up and out of the way.

Dressing for your bump

By the end of the second trimester you will probably have a bump of some sort to have to dress for.

Every woman is different and as a result bump sizes and shapes can also differ.

I had a very noticeable bump by around 16 weeks but had begun feeling clothes tightening due to bloating many weeks before.

Knowing that I was only going to get bigger I picked up a few tips along the way on dressing on a budget.

Luckily we now live in an age where maternity clothes are found in most of our high street shops. However, if you're already living on a budget investing in a new temporary wardrobe can be an unwanted expense.

Fear not there are things you can do to help make your current wardrobe last longer.

1. Make sure you know what's in your wardrobe, chances are you might have a pair of trousers in a size or 2 up. Failing that you might have tops or trousers with a little give or stretch. Dresses with the waist clinching belts, may be wearable without the belts. Long shirts that were worn as dresses may be able to be worn with a few buttons undone and a pair of leggings.

2. If you've got long tops to wear over trousers, leave the trousers undone. To prevent them falling down use an elastic band or hairband for a longer extension. For extra protection you might need a safety pin alongside your elastic. You can also shell out on a Bella Band which is basically a band that goes over your bump and trousers to help hide the fact they are unbuttoned and add extra support. I found an old tube top that did near enough the same thing though for half the price.

3. As mentioned in the first trimester section your breasts will change throughout the whole pregnancy. Until you need to change your bra, don't. It may be just as comfortable to buy a bra extender which you can find for a lot cheaper than a maternity bra.

Inevitably this may not work for all of us and in the end you may need to shell out on some items to get you through.

Here's some tips to get you through:

1. Buy the basics! – New look does an excellent basic starter pack for maternity. It had a baby bump band, a vest top and a pair of maternity leggings. I still use the vest top and leggings, now 3 months after labour. The vest top is long enough to cover any bulges as well as supportive of my nursing breasts.

2. Invest in a pair of maternity trousers for work and a pair of maternity skinny jeans. Both items can be dressed up or down for a variety of occasions. I recommend either New Look or H&M's ranges. There are mainly 2 types of jean, over the bump or under the bump. It's whatever feels more comfortable. I found over the bump made me feel more supported especially as my core muscles were so weak (due to a lack of fitness). I think it may also depend on how your carrying

3. Accessorise! – You may not have an extensive wardrobe during pregnancy but you can accessorise to add variety. The likes of Primark or Forever 21 have excellent accessory sections at affordable prices.

4. Don't be afraid to hit the internet. With most of us resorting to online shopping don't forget about the hidden gems. I bought a load of my maternity and baby stuff off of EBay. ASOS also have an excellent maternity range and I believe New Look items also appear onsite.

Finally, don't be afraid to buy more affordable items non maternity. It may be that a larger size in an affordable style may be more figure flattering. The word maternity automatically adds a premium in most shops.

Before you go overboard though just remember pregnancy doesn't last forever but that doesn't mean you have to look frumpy and unfashionable either.

New born baby checklist

By the end of the second trimester I was beginning to worry about how I was going to afford everything the baby might need. I also wanted to make sure I had everything prepared for her arrival in advance.

A little each month will end up being a lot more affordable than trying to buy it all off of one payslip.

Below you'll find a list of items that are essential as well as some added extras.

- Nappies – whether reusable or disposable, babies go through a hell of a lot of nappies up to 12 a day. Be aware though that they also grow very fast. I ended up buying a few boxes in the first 3 sizes just to get me started. You don't know how big or small the baby is going to be and you don't want to waste them.

- Nappy Cream – This can help prevent and treat nappy rash and irritation

If buying disposable make sure you take advantage of the offers available in store. Supermarkets regularly have offers on both nappies and baby wipes. I personally found Pampers to be the best for both nappies and wipes but the other brands may work better for you. Amazon also have an excellent offer sometimes and if buying in advance you can take advantage of the Free Super Saver delivery. Even up to now I order my nappies and wipes off of Amazon. It may only seem like a few pounds saving but on SMP those few pounds quickly add up.

- Three or four all in ones with sleeves. These tend to be able to be bought in packs. In most shops they come in at least a pack of 3. They will have sleeves and poppers underneath. Most babies tend to live in these for at least the first few months. Again I bought these in a few different sizes to make sure I had items in advance of when I'd need them.

- Three or four vests. These are similar to the all in ones but don't have sleeves. They tend to be worn underneath an all in one or outfit. When really hot or at home your baby may be comfortable in just a vest and socks.

Most supermarkets now have clothing ranges so it may be an idea to pick up a packet or two as part of your monthly or weekly food shop. The color range does tend to be limited though with white, beige, blue and pink available. You can also check out the likes of EBAY for second hand (or new with tags) bundles at a variety of sizes.

- A baby bath or New born bath support. The baby bath tends to be a size that the baby can actually go into filled with water. The new born bath support may be a chair type design that goes into your normal bath. There are also top and bottom bath units which you fill with water and clean the baby, without actually putting the baby into it. They are called top and bottom bath units because they have separate sections for the water for the face (top) and bottom of the baby. I ended up buying both but in fairness I could have just as easily used a washing up bowl from the pound store.

- Hooded soft towels – these are not only cute but help keep baby warm once their hair gets wet.

- Baby bath soap – You will be advised not to use any products with chemicals in them for at least the first few weeks. Sumaya ended up being allergic to one of the well-known brands so I have had to revert to Oilatum which has cleared up all dry skin. This is available on prescription but that was once her dry skin had already developed. I had previously ignored Oilatum in the shops as one with no cute baby smell but it is definitely kinder and more moisturising for her skin. In fairness I could have and should have purchased it before she was born.

- Bottles, teats, steriliser unit if you decide to bottle feed. You may also want one of these if you are planning on breastfeeding but will want to express. An expressing unit either manual unit or electrical may come with a bottle and steriliser – the Tommee Tippee one did anyway.

- Pram/Pushchair/Travel System – Be sure to try out the one you are interested in for usability. You will end up needing a car seat to take the baby home from the hospital (even if you don't have a car) so it may be an idea to buy one that comes with it.

- Moses basket or cot – You will be advised not to use a duvet until the baby is older, so stick to cellular blankets and cot sheets

- One or two cardigans and out layers to add an extra layer of warmth.

- Cotton wool/Cotton pads/Cotton Buds – These can be used for nappy changing or cleaning

- Muslin Squares – You honestly cannot have enough of these. I had about 20 but even that's not enough and I find myself wishing we had more. They have so many uses, cleaning baby during bath time, mopping up sick, feeding times, and resting babies head on.

- Nursing bras and breast pads – if you're planning on breastfeeding these will be a godsend. Breasts really do leak sometimes even when thinking about your baby.

- Milk Storage containers – I wish this had been on my list, I didn't think about what I'd store expressed milk in once I expressed it. I prefer the containers similar to a freezer bag. Reason being – you can easily label them and store up to 12 Oz per container.

- Snowsuit – If your baby happens to be born in winter you'll want the extra layer of warmth for taking them outside. Even if you plan on staying in during the winter you may still want to have one on hand.

- Scratch mittens and baby socks – Mittens are not really used to keep babies hands warm but more to stop the baby scratching their face. I put socks in the same line because I ended up using socks on Sumaya's hands because they weren't as easy for her to get off as the mittens

- New born hats – Most outfits come with a matching hat, but it's best to have a few on hand. Babies lose heat through their heads so to keep them warm the hats are important

- Healthcare/Grooming Kit – This consists of a thermometer, baby scissors, bulb syringe (to take the bogey out of baby's nose), emery boards (nail files), nail clippers, baby comb and brush – By all means you can buy the items individually but I purchased them in a set. It was definitely more cost efficient.

o Baby Monitor – When in another room you can have your baby monitor attached to your clothes or in a pocket. They enable you to hear (and sometimes see depending on the model) your baby and communicate with them. It may be that your baby needs to hear your voice to reassure them you are on your way. It's an added sense of comfort.

Non-Essential Items

o Changing table - You can purchase these as a matching unit to most cots. There are also cot top changers that attach to the top of your cot. Alternatively you may just buy a changing mat for use on any surface

o Rocking Chair - This was the one item I promised myself pre pregnancy. It is particularly useful if you plan on breastfeeding. You spend a lot of your time in the first few months breastfeeding so you may as well be comfortable.

o Sling/Baby Carrier – These are useful both in the house and out. They enable you to have your hands free and do tasks while at home. Babies are said to be more content close to their parent so these come in very handy. I made the huge mistake of not testing out my chosen carrier with a weighted doll before she was born. I ended up having a very complicated Sling which has not yet been used due to its complexity.

o Changing Bag – Some travel systems come with these but you may want to purchase one if it doesn't. They have many sections for the various items baby will need on journeys out. Most also come with a matching changing mat and sometimes a bottle holder.

- Baby sensory mat – Some baby monitor systems come with a sensor mat. They are basically a sensor that goes under the baby mattress. If they detect an issue with the baby's breathing an alarm will sound.

- Car Starter Set – If you're a driver you may want to purchase a baby on board sign with sun shades for the windows.

- Baby rattles/toys – There isn't many toys that a new born will even notice at such a young age. You can always buy in advance if you have the space for storage. For the meantime mirrors, rattles, and toys with different textures will do. Remember the baby has been in your womb for its entire life, the whole world is like a massive sensory playground.

- Baby bouncer – These are chairs for the baby to sit in. In terms of cost, they vary widely. Whichever one you choose ensure they are suitable for your new born. If cost is not an issue you may want to look into the 4moms Mamaroo.

- Nightlight – Some mums swear by night lights/sleep trainers. These play sounds that your baby may have heard when in the womb to add a sense of comfort and reassurance. If you decide to purchase they come in many different shapes and sizes from Little stars to Ewan the sheep.

- Dummy's – There are many different opinions on the use of dummys/pacifiers. If you choose to use one it may be an idea to have more than one on hand. Be sure to purchase ones suitable for a new born.

The Second Trimester summed up

As I said, the second trimester was my favourite part of pregnancy. I remember the first kick or punch from Sumaya inside my womb. It was a shock initially and then quite exciting. Initially only I could feel them and that added to the fact that I was and am her mum. The bond between mother and child is established long before the birth.

Whether you realise it or not yet, you are a very special being.

You're the protector and nurturer of this unborn child and as she or he moves around they remind you of exactly how special you are, to them at least.

One thing I wish we had done though is get away. With this being the most settled time of the pregnancy it was the perfect opportunity to get away. That doesn't necessarily mean flying away it could be a trip to a nice B&B or hotel in a different town or city. Alternatively you can stay at home, whether with a partner or on your own you can have some relaxation time.

Before long it will be all babies and feeding schedules so it's important to fit in some 'YOU' time.

The last trimester is definitely focused on the upcoming birth and parenthood so be sure to enjoy the excitement of pregnancy in this trimester. Shopping for your maternity wardrobe and then shopping for your new born essentials it's a trimester of enjoyment and excitement.

6 - 9 Months – Third Trimester

You're on the home straight! For some that's excitement, for others relief, for many it's fear.

The third trimester is definitely a time to plan and understand the upcoming labour and delivery.

Your stomach is probably very well rounded by now but your baby has a lot more growing to do in these last 3 months. As a result your stomach is going to get a whole lot bigger too.

You will be feeling a lot of movement from baby especially at the beginning of this trimester with the baby growing from approximately 37cm to 51cm by birth.

This is a trimester full of midwife appointments and antenatal classes resulting in information overload.

Be excited though, and enjoy it – Baby is on its way Mummy!!

Changes to your body

Baby Bump

Your stomach may be rounded by now and either high or low depending on how you're carrying.

There is an old wives tale that talks about the way you're carrying determining your baby's gender but there is absolutely no proof to that to be honest. I spent a lot of time prior to my anomaly scan trying to guess the gender of my baby. I was right 50% of the time lool... it was really a waste of time but I've always been pretty impatient.

Towards the end of the trimester in the run up to labour your stomach will 'drop'. I didn't know what everyone was talking about when they would ask 'has your stomach dropped yet?'

I didn't realise they literally meant my bump dropping. I was already carrying quite low anyway but towards the 6th and 7th month I still could feel Sumaya's feet by what I presume was my rib cage. At times I would literally feel winded and bruised from the inside.

When my bump began to drop there was a lot more pressure between my thighs. It genuinely felt like I had a basketball in between my legs that I was trying to keep up. I thought if I sneezed too hard she'd come shooting out and across the floor.

The baby dropping is actually known as lightening. In a first time pregnancy this can happen 3-4 weeks before labour and although it's a step in the right direction it doesn't give any indication of when labour will begin. There is less pressure on your stomach which should relieve some of that horrible heartburn you've likely been suffering with. If you've been getting breathless that should ease up too as your lungs will have more room.

Throughout the trimester though try to remember to moisturise your bump with Bio Oil or Cocoa Butter. With such rapid growth you may develop stretch marks even if you have been mark free up till now. Massaging the bump may also help you and your partner to bond with the baby.

If you're lucky, and your baby is being cooperative you might even get a kick or elbow.

<u>Breast preparation</u>

As mentioned previously your breasts will continue to grow as your belly does. I think for me the biggest growth spurt for my breasts during pregnancy was in the third trimester.

Most noticeable for me in this trimester though was how heavy they became.

Your breasts begin to produce colostrum in the run up to labour and birth in preparation to your baby. In some cases you may even feel the need to wear a breast pad.

I hadn't read up about colostrum or breast leakage as I presumed it would only happen after she was actually born. I recall one morning in the shower I noticed what I thought were scabs on my nipples. I had absolutely no idea if they had always been there or if they were another of the things that happen to women during pregnancy. It wasn't until I tried to pick at them that I realised the so called scabs were coming off in the shower and were wet. It was then that I reverted to google and realised I had begun producing colostrum.

Some woman begin leaking colostrum as early as their second trimester but for many it's towards the end that it's most noticeable.

Colostrum is a yellowish liquid sometimes known as liquid gold. It's full of all the antibodies needed to protect a new born baby from the bacteria and viruses of the world.

Don't be concerned if your leaking it though, once your baby is delivered it reproduces it and you will make some more. It's particularly important for a new born as it helps them pass their first stools also known as meconium. More about that in our labour and delivery section.

Pelvic Girdle Pain or Symphysis Pubic Dysfunction

In the same way I was plagued with round ligament pain in trimester one, I was hit with SPD in trimester 3.

Symphysis Pubic Dysfunction is a common complaint of many women in pregnancy sometimes known as Pregnancy Pelvic Girdle Pain. This is where the pelvic joints misaligns. It can (and did for me) cause severe pain around your pelvic area and pubic bone. Even worse for some it can cause pain by your perineum (area between vagina and anus) and across your lower back. For most this will lead to pain along your thighs.

There are a number of different reasons why SPD affects some women (about 1 in 5 pregnancies). Mainly it's to do with the weight and position of the baby. If you've had previous pelvic issues this will also increase your risk of developing it too.

The pain got a lot worse when I was walking, particularly going up or down the stairs and getting in and out of bed. I would literally be in tears with pain and would need my partner to put my leggings on, one leg at a time. At times when he wasn't around I would have to sit down to put on my leggings or shoes, slowly. It seemed that any movement involving the legs being separated caused excruciating pain. There is only so many things you can do where you don't separate your legs.

There are a number of things you can do to reduce your pain though.

- Keeping your knees together when turning over in bed – this was a lifesaver for me. I'd use this method when getting in and out of bed too. Knees closed and roll
- Pillow in between your knees when laying down – the comfort you will get from this even if you don't have SPD is almost orgasmic!
- Resting whenever possible
- Take the stairs one at a time
- If you feel up to a little intimate time find a position that's comfortable – all fours might work

One thing that really, really worked for me (yes I intentionally doubled up my really's) is a belly band. I did buy an expensive one off of EBAY specifically for SPD but this was a big clunky unattractive thing that could be seen through my clothes and didn't really help.

What I did end up using is the belly band purchased as part of the maternity starter kit from New Look. The basic band supported the weight of my bump and made me feel comforted. I believe it was the additional support that enabled me to still be able to walk around because without it I was in agony.

I promise you though, you will find ways to do things, it may look strange and you may feel a little embarrassed but people now days are used to seeing pregnancy women doing crazy things so it's nothing new. Embrace it!

If it gets really bad though or if you want it confirmed do mention it to your midwife at your earliest antenatal appointment. You may be offered a referral to a physiotherapist.

Most NHS Physiotherapy departments have specially trained physiotherapists for pelvic pain in pregnancy. Physiotherapy lessons may include manual therapy to make sure you have as much movement as possible.

They will show you pelvic floor and stomach exercises to strength your pelvis both during pregnancy and after delivery. You may also be given advice specific for a woman with SPD on labour and birth. **Labour with SPD -** I will go into a lot more detail on labour towards the end of this section but I would like to note SPD does not prohibit you having a vaginal birth as normal. You will want to note this in your birth plan though so that those involved in your labour can support you appropriately.

You may also want to think about different positions that are comfortable for you to give birth in. A water birth may be an option as this should take the weight off of your joints. If a water birth is not an option there are plenty of labour positions available.

Braxton Hicks contractions

Braxton Hick Contractions are the tightening of your womb. If you had your hands over your stomach when one happens you will feel your bump go hard.

They don't last very long and shouldn't cause any pain or discomfort.

Some women feel these as earlier as the second trimester but your womb will have been tightening since very early on in the pregnancy. I think you notice these more in later pregnancy because your uterus is bigger and you're more in tune with all the pregnancy niggles.

Towards the end of pregnancy in the third trimester and definitely in the run up to labour the Braxton hicks will become more intense and sometimes even painful. They act as an excellent practice run for the breathing techniques you plan on using in labour.

Braxton Hicks may even be confused with the real thing but when resting should ease off if not disappear altogether. Sometimes people refer to them as false labour pains for how similar they are. Below is a list of how to distinguish between a Braxton Hick (sometimes called a BH for short) versus a real labour contraction:

Braxton Hicks:

- Are usually not painful
- Do not happen at regular intervals – i.e. every 5 mins
- Do not get closer together
- Do not increase with movement i.e. walking around
- Do not feel stronger as they go on
- Do not last long – usually less than a minute

If you are experiencing pain with them though you should try to rest and see if they go away. Alternatively a change in activity might help i.e. sitting down if you've been standing up, or walking around if you've been sitting down etc. Warmth can also help so a warm bath should make them disappear or decrease.

Antenatal appointments

In this trimester the number of antenatal appointments will increase.

By 31 weeks you will be having an appointment every 2 weeks. For the most part providing there are no complications they will follow a very similar pattern

With your anomaly scan now done, if it doesn't require any follow up your scans are all done for this pregnancy. This doesn't mean they aren't checking on baby though they just use other methods.

If they haven't already they will be listening to your baby's heartbeat at each appointment using a fetal heart Doppler. This is a hand held device that measures your baby's heartbeat. They put some gel (the same as when they do a scan) and move the device around your bump until they pick up the heartbeat.

Many woman compare the sound to galloping horses or the sound of a train. The heartbeat should be somewhere in the range of 120 – 160 beats per minute.

A faster or slower beat than this may indicate a problem. When concerned your midwife may send you to the OAU at your local hospital. Obstetrics Assessment Units will likely place you on a monitor for up to an hour to get a print out of your baby's heartbeat. This is similar to the Doppler except the plates used to pick up the heartbeat are held in place with belly bands. The report is then analysed and checked by a doctor.

You will also have your urine tested for protein and blood pressure checked as normal. Any indications of preeclampsia or gestational diabetes will be followed up and investigated.

Your iron levels will be checked and if found to be low you will be advised to take iron levels. I ended up having low iron levels which were contributing to my tiredness. They were actually on the line of being too low but I was advised to take them anyway and ended up feeling much better.

Iron is needed to help our red blood cells carry oxygen around our bodies. Almost 25% of pregnant women end up with iron-deficiency in pregnancy. Iron deficiency is classed as being under 11g per DL of blood. Mine were 15g per DL but with the tablets went up to 120g.

The only negative I found with the iron tablets was the constipation it caused. To combat that I just had to increase my fruit and veg intake which had its additional benefits for me and baby.

Additionally your bump will start being measured. This is literally a measurement of your bump from the top of your womb to the bottom by your pubic hair.

The measurement should be close to the number of weeks you are. I was fascinated by this, I was always 1cm out, so at 31 weeks my bump was measuring around 30cm etc. In the end Sumaya ended up being almost exactly a week late. The midwife would have a little feel of my bump and sometimes indicate which bits were where.

I would urge you to keep notes of any question you have for your midwife though. It's a really good opportunity to ask anything you have had on your mind. Most midwifes are really kind and all are qualified in answering your questions or referring you to someone that can.

Birthing Plan

At some point during your third trimester you will be asked about your birth plan. I ended up doing this myself beforehand but the midwife was on hand to answer any additional questions I had.

Your birth plan is made by you, with any input you need from your midwife and any Parentcraft sessions you have attended.

The basis of a birth plan is as below.

- Where you intend on giving birth
- Who you intend on being at the birth with you
- Whether you would want your birth partner/s in the room if medical interventions are required i.e. forceps delivery or caesarean
- What birthing equipment you intend on using
- How often you want the baby monitored during labour

- How active you want to be during labour
- The positions you want to try during labour
- Any conditions that may affect your labour – such as SPD etc.
- Once delivered where you want the baby placed
- Whether a student can be involved in your labour
- The pain relief you want to try
- Whether you understand what an episiotomy is and why you might need one
- Who you would like to cut the cord
- How you want the placenta delivered
- Whether you want the baby to have the Vitamin K shot
- How you plan on feeding the baby
- If you have any special requirements for delivery or you're new born.

It is important to note though that most women will say they didn't end up following their birth plan and for me that was also the case.

However what it did do was help me to feel informed about the choices I made. My intention was to follow the plan but when it came down to it I completely forgot what I wanted and just wanted Sumaya out.

Also during your antenatal appointment your midwife will want to make sure you are in good health, with normal fetal movement and minimal pain.

They will advise you to go to the delivery suite if you have: decreased fetal movement, contraction pain or vaginal bleeding.

During this trimester you should also be advised on the antenatal classes available in your area.

These may also be known as parent craft classes.

ParentCraft classes (antenatal classes) – NHS

I am unsure about how other NHS hospitals run their classes but I presume the content is somewhat similar. This section will both describe the classes (run over 4 sessions) as well as fill you in on what I learnt about preparing for labour.

There were 4 sessions for my antenatal classes. They tend to run throughout the week at set times and also on the weekends which is useful if you or your partner are working.

The class titles were as followed

1.   Normal birth and pain relief

2.   Variation of labour and birth

3.   Postnatal care, Postnatal depression

4.   Infant feeding and tour of delivery suite.

I presume that the ParentCraft classes are as good as the midwife running them as well as the people attending. If both are communicative the classes will not only be informative but enjoyable too.

Other than ParentCraft lessons you can pay for antenatal classes outside of the NHS.

The most known and most highly rated is the NCT classes.

NCT Classes

NCT (National Childbirth Trust) run a number of different courses and workshops to prepare you for both childbirth and parenthood. They explore both the practical and emotional changes you are likely to experience.

You fill in a form registering your interest and someone from your local NCT team will contact you to discuss your requirements as well as inform you of local courses available to you.

Many use the NCT to meet other parents in their area. The NHS classes tend to have different people in them and there isn't the closeness a smaller group can provide.

I have heard many great reviews about the NCT classes both from the internet and new parents.

From what I understand many continue their friendships after the courses have finished meeting for coffee mornings etc.

For more information you can look on the NCT website. **www.nct.orguk**

Everything I know about Labour

As pregnant woman approaching labour there are many questions about concerns associated with how you're going to get this baby out. Not only that but you also may want to know how you'll know you're in labour.

Will it be like on the TV with water gushing everywhere and then you have to push?

Will you be doing the food shop and your water breaks in Asda? If so, will they call you an ambulance or a cab?

As with everything labour is a unique experience for each woman, and each pregnancy. I should probably tell you about my experience while I go into the details.

My EDD was the 3rd February 2014. I expected to go into labour beforehand and had no plans to be overdue. The 3rd Feb came and went and nothing happened, disappointed wasn't the word. I had read that most 1st time mums will be overdue but I hadn't thought that included me. So the 3rd Feb 14, is a Monday and my antenatal appointments always fell on a Thursday. On the Thursday there was still no baby so I was offered a membrane sweep.

A membrane sweep is where the midwife/doctor puts a gloved finger inside your vagina up to your cervix. The aim of a membrane sweep is to separate the amniotic sac (which surrounds your baby) from your cervix. This is a form of induction and should help bring on labour. Now I had already researched before the appointment as I knew it would be something offered. I can honestly say I have never been so scared in my whole life. I spent the 4th and 5th researching ways to bring on labour naturally to prevent me having to get this sweep done.

Nothing is forced upon you in pregnancy though so I was under no obligation to have the sweep done. However, the fact that it was either this or a potential induction with drugs I knew I would have the sweep done if need be.
I sat there the night before the arranged sweep googling sentences.
'Does a sweep hurt?'
'Success rates of a sweep'
In answer to the question, I can talk from experience. Does a sweep hurt? – Well, ye it does, is the fair answer. However, does it hurt as much as you think it will? – No.
 It honestly was no more painful than a smear test. How long or how short the sweep is actually done for – in terms of duration, is up to you. If you say stop the midwife or doctor will stop. I actually just gritted my teeth and focused on the posters on the wall. I had my partner in the room and asked him to read the nearest poster to him and explain what it looked like in detail. In the end the midwife stopped of her own accord and said her hand was now hurting.

They do say that you should probably bring a pad to a sweep as there may be some bleeding and period like cramps. I had no bleeding but definitely could feel the cramps.

Your advised to continue with your natural induction methods with the hope that these and the sweep will mean labour is imminent.

The natural methods I found (some used, some not) included:

- Walking – vigorous as possible with a bump, a bit like power walking for as long as possible. Be careful not to tire yourself out though in case it works. Labour is tiring enough
- Stairs – Walking up and down stairs is said to help as your legs are apart and gravity can work its magic
- Raspberry Leaf Tea – this can be purchased from health food stores and can be bought in both teabag and tablet form
- Sex – Sexual intercourse is said to produce the hormone needed to kick start labour
- Bouncing on a birthing ball, literally bouncing in sitting position and doing figure 8's with your hips
- Spicy Food – be careful as this may add to you already painful heartburn
- Cinnamon stick tea – A whole cinnamon stick with water
- Squats – Wide legged squats help push baby into the birth canal
- Castor Oil – Really not recommended and not one I personally tried, has some really bad reviews and can lead to painful diarrhoea for you and baby

Before I left for home my midwife called the delivery suite to book me in for an induction for the following week in case I reached 41 + 5 without delivering.

An induction is normally booked to happen after 41 weeks pregnant.

This is where labour is started artificially. Although a membrane sweep is classed as a method of induction this may not actually work and is said to stimulate labour.

The other methods are more synthetic. With this a possibility I again went home to get clued up.

There are two main methods used. The first is a pessary, tablet or gel inserted into your vagina. This contains a hormone like substance called prostaglandin. This works by causing your cervix to ripen and therefore may stimulate contractions and start the whole labour process off. In some hospitals you will be able to go home and come back but for my area the policy is to be admitted and monitored.

This was therefore not a route I wanted to go down as part of my birth plan was to stay at home for as long as possible.

The other option if the prostaglandin didn't work was another synthetic form of a hormone but this time it was Syntocinon.

For this to be used it would have been administered via a drip and my waters would have to have been broken beforehand. I was also advised that I would probably need an epidural administered at the same time because the contractions from an induction are a lot more powerful.

As with most things there may also be a small risk of overstimulation of the uterus and a reduction of oxygen to the baby. This is why the baby and mum are monitored so closely.

The medical team are able to stop the induction and provide drugs to slow the contractions down so you shouldn't worry.

I came to the conclusion that if I needed to have an induction I was just going to have to accept it but really I would continue to try with all the natural methods and hope for the best.

While at home I begun to have really painful period like cramps. I knew it was as a result of the membrane sweep and hoped it would continue and lead on to labour.

I checked and doubled checked my hospital bag against the hospital checklist I'd compiled listing all the things I'd need while at the hospital.

This had been packed from around 34 weeks as I had presumed I would go into labour early.

Hospital Checklist:

This I split into two sections, a section for me and a section for baby

For **Mum:**

- o Nightdress/T Shirt to give birth in – labour is a very messy process so if you do buy one make sure it's not expensive. You will want to throw this item away once it's been used. Alternatively you can give birth in a hospital gown. If you're planning on having an epidural you will need to use the gown as your back has to be exposed.
- o Nightdress for after labour – in case it's at night and you want to sleep
- o Clothes to go home in – you will feel sore so something comfortable. I opted for maternity legs and a baggy jumper. Your stomach won't be round but you are unlikely to be flat either. You may feel bruised and will want something loose
- o Knickers – you can buy special disposable knickers

- Nursing Bra – you will want these in at least 1 size bigger, possibly two if you will be in hospital for a few days as your milk may come in
- Normal toiletries – soap, shampoo, deodorant, toothpaste, toothbrush, shampoo etc. I recommend the travel versions though so your bag isn't too big or heavy.
- Sanitary towels – you will have lochia (postnatal bleeding) which can be like a really heavy period so night time sanitary towels might be best
- Breast pads – even if you don't plan on breastfeeding you may still leak colostrum/milk
- Pillow – yes some hospitals don't have pillows available to use
- Mobile phone and charger
- Something to entertain you i.e. pregnancy book, pack of cards etc. – just because you're in established labour doesn't mean it will be a quick process. You may be bored until the baby actually comes
- Music – in some hospitals you can bring music in to play during labour. You may need the actual device to play the music though as one may not be provided.
- Hairbrush and bands – you'll want to tie our hair up if it's annoying during labour. Once the baby has arrived though you may want to brush your hair for photo's
- Lip Balm – labour wards tend to be warm which may dry out your lips
- Water spray – labour can make you really hot and sweaty so a birthing partner can lightly spray you with water to keep you cool.
- A flannel and towel – the small ones you can use to keep baby warm will not be enough to dry yourself after a shower.
- Dressing Gown – sometimes to speed up labour you might pace the corridors of the hospital. To hide stains or leakages you might want a dark coloured one.
- Snacks and water – you'll need energy bars/light snacks to get you through and for once you've finished.

For **Baby:**

- o Two or three vests (mentioned in earlier chapters) – remember you don't know what size baby will come out as so you might want a first size, 0 -3 and a new born one just in case
- o Two or three all in one sleep suits – same as above in terms of sizing
- o Baby blanket – you may want to have your own blanket to keep baby warm and may also need it when you head home
- o Disposable Nappies – Size 1 should be okay as it covers most birth weights. You may need up to 12 a day for a new born
- o Muslin squares – multi functional, these may come in handy for cleaning up baby and mopping up spit up
- o Socks- Baby's feet always feel cold even if they are relatively warm
- o Hat – Baby's lose heat from their heads and will definitely need a hat to leave
- o Mittens
- o One outfit for the trip home
- o Baby car seat – you are not allowed to leave the hospital without one
- o Snowsuit – if baby is born in the winter they will need one, otherwise a jacket should be enough

Once checked I figured I should get as much rest as possible. I presumed I would go into labour during the night and would therefore need all the sleep I could get.

The following morning came and went and still nothing. I sent my partner out for some more Cinnamon sticks and sat there popping the raspberry leaf pills from Holland and Barratt. I was still having the cramps but I hadn't yet experienced the tell-tale signs that labour had started.

Signs you've started labour

1. Abdominal pain with pre-menstrual like cramps – TICK
   Well I certainly had these and could easily distinguish them as I was a regular period pain sufferer pre pregnancy

2. The 'Show' – A bloody sometimes brownish discharge. It is sometimes referred to as mucus discharge because the discharge literally looks like mucus that comes out of your nose. For some woman it comes out as one blob but for me it had been passing from even before the membrane sweep in little dribs and drabs.

3. Broken Waters – This is unlikely to be as dramatic as you see on the TV but will be a gush of water. For some it may just be a continuous trickle of water. At the antenatal classes a woman asked a really good question. 'If I'm in the shower and pass my water's, how will I know?' The midwife advised that the waters won't stop. It will continue after you've gotten out of the shower. We were also asked to take note of its colour. Clear or a little Yellow = Good, Red or Green = Bad. Red being blood isn't a good sign so you'll need to get to hospital. Green means the baby has passed its meconium while inside (its first stools) and is at risk of infection. It's also important to note the delivery suite (if you're having the baby at the hospital/birthing centre) will want to know your waters have gone. Alternatively if you have opted for a home birth your home birth team will also need to know. They will want the baby delivered within 24 hours.

4. Contractions – Contractions are very difficult to describe and I also think they are different for every woman. Some say they are like worse versions of Braxton hicks others say they are like really bad period pains. For me I didn't really know I was experiencing contractions as they were a continuation from the cramps I had been feeling since the membrane sweep the day before.

5.   An upset stomach or loose bowels – This can be best described as clearing your body out in preparation for birth.

So I had the cramps which I didn't think were contractions until I actually delivered Sumaya and realised they must have been. My mucus plug was coming away and I had an upset stomach but this could have been attributed to food intake and the membrane sweep. In hindsight though I was in the latent phase of labour and just didn't know it.

Stages of labour

Labour is split into 3 stages.

The first stage is usually the longest and is sometimes known as the latent phase. This is when the contractions make your cervix open (gradually). You need to get to 10cm dilated for a baby to be able to pass through. You won't be in established labour until your cervix has dilated more than 3cm.

I was in this latent phase, without being in established labour for approximately 34 hours. I learnt one important lesson though – do not go into the hospital until you're in established labour – you will be sent home. Throughout the Friday (the day after the sweep) I was still having these period type pains but since I hadn't experienced contractions before I didn't know if they were contractions.

To be fair I didn't know what they were all I knew is they would come, reach a maximum intensity and then slow down, eventually disappearing. I can best describe it like riding a bike up a hill, reaching the top out of breath before gliding back towards the bottom and the rest point. Since they lasted for so long, 34 hours in total before I reached established labour I was able to test out and rotate different coping mechanisms.

Coping Mechanisms

During the latent phase before you're in established labour there are many things you can try since you will most likely be at home.

One thing that really helped me was understanding that each contraction will only last for a period of time. It isn't like they are continuous. You do get a break in between. Deal with one contraction at a time and don't think about how long you have left or how many more you have to go until it's over.

Every contraction gets you closer to the end result of your baby being born.

In the meantime here are my tips on coping:

- Breathing – Breathing is probably the best and most effective coping mechanism for all contractions. It's hard to explain but there is a different type of breathing that can help you get through each contraction. A tip I picked up in one of the forums was to think about the word RELAX. Make the RE part quick and the LAX bit long. RELAAAAXXXXXXX. Now change that into breathing. Quick breath in = RE, long breath out = LAX. Pass this on to your birth partner/s to remind you during labour. It also helps if they do it with you so you might want to practice beforehand.

- Relax – the likelihood is you'll be in the latent phase of labour for a long time so do you best to relax. Whether that means watching a film, going for a walk, try to take your mind off of it. At the same time though don't use up too much energy as you will need that for later on.

- Take a warm bath or shower – for me this really helped. It didn't necessarily take the pain away but helped relax me and as a result I felt more able to cope. Getting out of the shower into the cold didn't feel very nice though so I'd quickly (as quickly as a pregnant person can move anyway) get back in.

- Have something to eat – In early labour you may feel hungry and if so try to have something to eat, this will help build up energy for the second stage of labour. I unfortunately was really sick and unable to keep anything down including water but I still tried whenever possible

- Try out different positions – now is an excellent time to try out new positions to give birth in since the pain won't be as intense. You may find rocking back and forth helps you to feel more comfortable. For back pain being on all fours really helped me. There are a number of different positions that can be tried out:

- Laying down with legs open
- All fours
- Standing
- Squatting
- Sitting on a birthing stool

- TENS machine- Ohh my favourite thing in the whole labour world. This is a device that is recommended by many midwifes. It isn't normally available to use at the hospital so if you want to use one you will have to bring your own. It is a machine with pads that go on your back. There are four pads, two that go near your bra clasp and two that go on your lower back. The idea is that the electric shocks stop your brain registering pain. Once the pain had continued for 12 hours I got my partner to put on my pads and hooked myself up to the TENS machine. These can be purchased outright or rented. Purchases can be bought off of the internet and may be available on the likes of EBAY or Amazon. If you're going to get a second hand one you will need new pads. If you're going to rent one, you should be able to from the likes of Argos, Boots, and Mothercare etc. I fell in love with the sensation of the electric shocks during the contractions. There was even a boost button for when the contraction reached its maximum intensity. For some woman it really helps and can be used up to the point of the second stage of labour. Others say it made no difference. For me it definitely helped, both in reducing the pain and in making me feel like I was doing something. Sometimes in labour you need something to focus on and the TENS definitely did that. Unfortunately I was in non-established labour for so long that the pads lost their stickiness and I didn't have any spare. It wasn't until I had to take off the machine that I realised how much it had been helping.

You're advised not to go to the hospital until you're in established labour of 3cm + dilated. As a result during your antenatal classes you're given tell-tale signs to look out for. Imagine if women had to check their own cervix!

Contractions are regular, strong, 5 minutes apart and lasting about 60 seconds each. This has to have been going on for about an hour.

To be honest, you will know when it's time to get to hospital. I had been sent home twice but that was mainly due to me wanting to confirm I was actually in labour. The time I got admitted I really knew it was time to go into hospital.
I had been at the hospital twice and each time was still only 1cm dilated. I couldn't believe it, I was unable to sleep properly through the contraction type pains although I had been resting.

As mentioned before I also couldn't eat without everything being brought back up. I was reaching the end of my tether and went into the shower and prayed. I literally scream prayed begging God to let this baby come now pleeeaassseee.

Within a few minutes I turned to my partner and said, "It's time!"

Now, remember I had dragged us down the hospital twice and each time we had been sent home. By now he had just left the hospital bags in the car refusing to bring them back upstairs into our flat. He said we should wait a few more hours and if my waters still hadn't broken then yes he would drive me back to the hospital.

That's an important note to make, it's best to check your chosen birth place for parking restrictions. Luckily my hospital has parking available but most hospitals don't. It may be an idea to find out which local cab firms are labour friendly. This is also an additional reason to go to the hospital at the point you believe you're in established labour. Traipsing back and forth to the hospital will not only be inconvenient and costly, it is also known to slow labour down.

Something in me knew that we wouldn't have a few more hours. I was fully prepared to beg the hospital staff to let me stay even if it meant getting a loan out and paying for a private room.

When we arrived at the delivery suite the process followed the same as the other 2 times I had been there.

- You check in with your folder (by now your pregnancy folder should be with you at all times in your handbag)

- You are seen by a first midwife who checks your blood pressure, pulse, temperature and abdomen (for baby's positioning). They may also record the baby's heartbeat (using a portable Fetal Doppler like the one the midwife uses at your antenatal appointments). You're also asked about why you're here i.e. frequency of contractions etc.

- If not already in a large enough room you may be taken into a side room or small ward to have an internal examination performed. This will let the midwife know how many cm's dilated you are

If you're in established labour you will be transferred to the delivery suite or birthing centre.

The birth centre is only run by midwives and there are no doctors. Depending on your pregnancy and chosen pain relief depends on whether you can have the baby in the birth centre.

Birthing centres are more comfortable and tend to be larger. They may have a wide range of equipment such as birthing stools, birthing pools, balls etc. Some hospitals may have a birthing centre connected to the delivery suite, so if a complication arises you can easily be transferred to the delivery suite. Other birthing centres may be away from the hospital and require an ambulance to transfer you. Your midwife will be able to confirm if a birth centre is an option available to you.

The delivery suite has a bed and chairs as you would imagine in a hospital environment. There may also be birthing pools and bean bags. Most delivery suites have their own en suite. They aim to make you as comfortable as possible both during and after labour.

As part of your Parentcraft classes there should be a tour of the delivery suite so you are familiar with what to expect. If this is not something available you should be able to call the delivery suite to arrange a tour.

My plan had been to take advantage of the birth centre connected to the delivery suite as I had planned to have minimal pain relief and rely on gas and air and the birthing pool. I was advised due to my increased BMI at the beginning of labour I would not be able to use the birth centre. At this point I honestly didn't really care and just wanted to be admitted. I felt exhausted and wanted to be given something to go to sleep. At this point it had taken 34 hours to actually be classed as being in established labour and I had had no sleep. To say I wasn't a happy bunny is an understatement.

I was shown into the OAU (Obstetric Assessment Unit) for my internal examination. Both the baby's heartbeat and my contractions were being monitored on a computer which printed out a report. It was reassuring and a spirit lifter to hear the baby's heartbeat. I may have been in pain and had had enough but she was oblivious.

A student midwife asked if she could check my cervix before the qualified midwife for her training. I had marked on my birth plan that I didn't really mind and I stuck by that. I figured she needed to learn and allowed her to check me. The qualified midwife then checked me and asked the student for her findings. She begun to smile at which point I was planning on what to say to get myself admitted.
I was convinced I would be sent home again but she said she thought I was 5cm. The qualified midwife confirmed this to be the case and I burst into tears. I was so excited that things had moved on and I would finally be going to the delivery suite.

They went off to find me a room and porter and left me to consider what pain relief I wanted.

Pain relief options in Labour

- **Water** is often used to relieve pain either in a birthing pool or simply a bath. This works in keeping you relaxed and helping you to focus on your breathing

- **Gas and Air (Entonox)** this is available both in the birth centre and delivery suite. You breathe in the air through a mouthpiece reducing the pain. It's important to note though it takes up to 20 seconds to work so it might take a little practise to get the timing right. It can make you feel light-headed or nauseous. The main positive of this though is you can stop using it if you don't like how it makes you feel.

- **Pethidine** is an injection normally administered into the thigh or bum cheek it acts as a pain killer. Some hospitals use diamorphine instead. It starts working approximately 20 mins after its administered but again can make you feel nauseous. Sometimes it can affect a woman's ability to push. If given too close to delivery it can also affect a baby's breathing (a drug is available to reverse this though). It can also affect a baby's first feed

- **Epidurals** are classed as a type of local anaesthetic. They numb the nerve blocking the brain from registering pain. It provides good pain relief but it's not always 100% effective. I believe it's around the 80% mark. This can only be administered by an anaesthetists so tends to only be available in the delivery suite. A thin needle is used to put a tube into your back. Once this is set up the epidural can be topped up by a midwife but the initial epidural is administered by the anaesthetist. You will have to have complete monitoring of the baby's heartbeat which will mean the belt around our abdomen. For many the epidural can make your legs numb. It can also give you a headache and in some cases your back will be a little sore for a few days after. The main issue with epidurals seem to be that it can make the second stage of labour more complicated as you may not be able to feel your contractions any longer. If this is the case you may not know when to push and may require instrumental delivery.

Instrumental delivery

An instrumental delivery is also known as assisted delivery. It's where forceps or a suction cup are used to help delivery the babies head. This may require an episiotomy to make the processes easier.

The suction cup is literally a cup attached to a machine that will pull the baby out. You will still need to push though. This may result in a small swelling or bruise on the baby's head but this will disappear. Your also less likely to tear with the suction cup method than the forceps.

Forceps delivery is with the use of metal instruments that look similar to tongs. Again you will need to push as the midwife pulls on the forceps (which will be placed around baby's head) to deliver the baby. This may result in small marks on the baby's face but again these are not permanent.

If the assisted delivery doesn't work or if the baby is lying in an awkward position you may need a caesarean.

Caesarean Delivery

Sometimes a caesarean may be required to deliver the baby. This may have been arranged beforehand (planned or elective caesarean) or come up during labour as an emergency.
Approximately 25% of babies in the UK are born this way.

A caesarean is a cut through into your womb just below your bikini line. It is classed as major surgery. You may be able to stay awake during the operation using an epidural. Sometimes though you will need to be put to sleep under general anaesthetic. The main disadvantage of going under general is that your birth partner will not be allowed to be in the operating theatre. You also won't see your baby until after you wake up.

You are allowed to choose to have a caesarean but you will need to discuss your reasons with the healthcare professionals. The risks involved with a caesarean are best avoided, especially if there is no medical need for a caesarean to be performed.

Such risks include:
- Infection to the womb or wound
- Excess bleeding
- Damage to your bladder.

The main reason I didn't want a caesarean is due to the recovery process being more difficult. It is a major operation with an actual wound. You are likely to stay in hospital for a few days after the birth.

Walking up and down stairs should be avoided in the first few weeks as you will still be sore. It is important to rest as much as possible with a newborn. You may require painkillers although check with your doctor and midwife if you are planning on breastfeeding.

It will take about 6 weeks until you begin to feel normal again. Take things at your own pace though and don't do anything if you don't feel up to it yet.

Once I had been shown into the delivery suite I settled onto the bed getting as comfortable as I could in between contractions. I was hooked onto the machine to monitor baby's heartbeat as the midwife had a quick read through my folder. She asked what pain relief options I had thought about and whether I wanted to discuss them.

Midwives are extremely patient human being's. I regularly had to stop midsentence to deal with another contraction. I was swapping and changing between using the RE..LAAXXXXX method of breathing to rainbow visualisation. I literally visualised myself walking up a steep rainbow which was where the contraction intensity increased, once at its peak I was at the top of the rainbow, this meant to everyone around me that they should not talk and let me concentrate. I then would say, 'sliding down the rainbow' which meant the pain was decreasing. During particularly bad contractions I would visualise a leprechaun waiting for me at the end as my rest spot. I don't even like leprechauns but it worked and helped me cope.
I had noted on my birth plan that I wanted to try gas and air as my main form of pain relief. The birth plan had been written prior to experiencing the lack of sleep so I decided I wanted whatever they could give me if it meant I could go to sleep. I was advised that the only thing that would take away the pain enough to let me sleep was an epidural. I remember replying 'That's what I'll have then'. I honestly wasn't interested in any other form of pain relief. It wasn't the pain as much as it was the tiredness.

It took a while for the anaesthetist to arrive as he was needed elsewhere. He went through the possible side effects of an epidural all of which I had previously read up on. He advised that he would put a starter epidural in first to make sure it was in the right place and then top it up with the rest.

To get into the correct position I had to sit with my legs off of the bed in a sort of slouched position exposing my back to him. You are advised not to move so if you have a contraction you have to let them know so they can stop.

As the starter epidural went in, I wet myself. I wish I could say it was my water breaking but it wasn't. Luckily I was already sitting on an absorbent pad so didn't make any mess. I then went into the second stage of labour.

The second stage of labour is the pushing stage. This happens when your cervix is fully dilated. This is the stage where you put in the work. It's hard work pushing a baby out but your midwife can help you find a position that's comfortable for you. It also helps to have a supportive birth partner cheering you on and encouraging you when you've had enough or feel like you've run out of steam.

I was waiting for the anaesthetist to come back with the rest of the epidural when I felt the urge to push. I'm still sitting up with my legs over the bed when I tell the midwife I needed to push. Remember I had been 5cm's approximately 20mins beforehand so it seemed unlikely that I was 10cm already.

I could see the disbelief on my partner and mum's face. I knew they didn't believe me but at that point it really didn't matter. I said 'I'm pushing'. The midwife said I shouldn't, because I was sitting up. Good point, I was pushing into the mattress.

I was checked internally – which I couldn't really feel to be honest. It was confirmed I really was 10cm. I wasn't paying much attention though because I was already pushing.

It honestly is an uncontrollable urge. You have no other option but to push. It didn't exactly feel pleasurable but I was pleased to be actually doing something. The first few pushes I don't think I was doing it right. You literally have to push into your bottom. It's a very strange sensation because you think you're going to go toilet (number 2). Some women do and I probably would have but there was nothing left to push out other than the baby.

You have to bear down and just push. The idea is not to make much noise i.e. screaming as this can make you push wrong. I ended up doing more of a grunt growl type noise. It is very hard work I can't lie and you feel like you're getting nowhere. Your asked to push through a contraction and then when you run out of breath take a quick breathe in and push again (providing the contraction hasn't ended). At this point the contractions are coming fast with little rest in between so you barely have time to catch your breath before you have to go again.

I was already laying down with my legs open. I tried the whole squeezing of my partners hand but that didn't work for me. I know my legs are a lot stronger than my upper body and ideally I would have wanted to squat to push her out but since this wasn't an option I was advised to put my feet into the leg holders and use them to push off of. It finally felt like I was getting somewhere.

During one of the breaks I could actually touch and feel her hair. I knew then that it was almost over but I was now dealing with a new anxiety. I didn't want to tear or have the cut.

Tearing in labour

Tearing in labour occurs between the vagina and anus at a site called the perineum. A tear is relatively common during childbirth.

There are four degrees of tearing

1st degree tear – tear is superficial, involving only skin around vagina. May sting when urinating but isn't severely painful

2nd degree tear – tear is slightly worse involving vagina and perineum. Requires stiches to repair.

3rd degree tear – tear involves vagina, perineum, and muscles around the anus. Requires repair in an operating theatre. Complicated 3rd degree tears may result in incontinence and painful intercourse

4th degree tear – most severe tear. Involve vagina, perineum, muscles around the anus and rectum lining. Will require operation and may take months to heal.

Sometimes an episiotomy will be performed to prevent a serious tear.

An episiotomy is a small diagonal cut from the back of the vagina backwards at an angle. This is done under local anaesthetic so you don't feel the pain. An episiotomy is also used to speed up birth if the baby is under distress or needs to come out quickly. The cut like a tear is stitched together using dissolvable stitches.

There can be some pain associated with tearing or an episiotomy for 2 to 3 weeks after the birth. The pain may increase when sitting or walking. Passing urine can also cause the area to sting. It is recommended to pour water over the area while urinating to take away the sting and provide a soothing sensation.

Some women also buy a doughnut-shaped cushion to sit on which is meant to relieve some of the pressure and therefore pain. You can also use icepacks to numb the area and relieve pain.

It is important to keep both the cut and tear area as clean as possible to prevent infection.

I had expressed my fears regarding tearing to my midwife and she had advised that I should maintain contact with the midwife delivering the baby. The idea is to listen to your midwife. If she says stop pushing it's for a reason.

As said, the urge to push is uncontrollable. However, I didn't want to tear and therefore when I was asked not to push to prevent tearing I panted like a dog and stopped pushing. This allowed the baby's head to emerge slowly giving my skin and muscles time to stretch without tearing.

The moment I was given the go ahead to push again though I pushed for dear life and out slid Sumaya – crying straight away. It was both extremely exciting yet extremely emotional. I was now officially someone's mummy.

As her daddy cut the ambilical cord I realized that this was now us. Whether we stayed together, split up, moved country, this would always be us. We were now all connected, mother, father and baby.

They placed Sumaya on my chest while they prepared for the aftercare and checks.

Not so yummy mummy after birth

Giving birth to a baby, a human being, a life is hard work. It puts your body under conditions that it hasn't previously had to deal with. Whether you've pushed the baby out or had a c-section having a baby is no joke. Once the baby is born, ye it was all worth it, but your body now has to recover and this takes some time.

Physically

If you have had a vaginal delivery you will feel really sore down there. I mean like really sore. Moving and walking is going to hurt, that's fact but it will get easier as the days pass. For many you will feel more uncomfortable after labour than you did during, particularly if you had strong pain relief such as an epidural.

You will bleed from your vagina after labour similar to a period. This is known as lochia and is similar to a really heavy period. This can continue for around 6 weeks although it will go from being heavy to light and annoying. I remember towards the end of the 6 weeks I'd think, 'hasn't this finished yet'. This may be associated with a little bit of period type cramps particularly when breastfeeding.

You should not use tampons as this increases the risk of infection. You should also pay close attention to make sure you are not passing blood clots larger than a 50 pence piece.

If you've got stiches from either an episiotomy or a tear the use of warm water can really help in relieving some pain or stinginess. I remember needing to drink loads of water to dilute my urine. I hadn't torn at all, but did have a very minor graze in my vaginal area that stung a little.

They also recommend using a bunch of clean tissues over the stiches when passing bowel movements just to keep the area clean. You're unlikely to open your bowels for a few days after birth. I remember being more scared about this than anything as it just felt lie it was going to hurt. I wasn't wrong….I got a bad case of piles after delivery. Apparently it's really common but that added absolutely no comfort.

The piles were unexpected but I did expect to bleed heavily and I did expect to be sore. What I didn't expect or consider though is how my stomach would react to the change. I don't know if I expected it to just be flatter than it was pre pregnancy or look bloated. I had no idea and couldn't visualize it. What I got was a shocker.

Your belly will be baggy…I know… baggy. It just doesn't sound right. So the baby has been born and the placenta delivered but you're left with the excess skin. It was strange to put a top on after Sumaya had been born. She looked so cute and I felt so uncomfortable. Gone was the bump, making my larger frame more acceptable. That's why I recommend the large baggy top.

Not only will your stomach look unattractive it may also feel really bruised. I felt like I had been run over by a car and then a van followed by a large double decker bus – twice. This is mainly due to the stretched muscles. Your body is working hard to get everything back in place.

Breastfeeding helps to bring your stomach down quite fast though. Breastfeeding causes your womb to contract which helps the stomach tone up. These contractions will hurt slightly though and may make the lochia heavier and more red in colour.

Speaking of breasts, oh my goodness – when your milk comes in!

By day 5 your breasts will be super tender as the milk comes in. I woke up and was like 'what the hell is going on now!' I was in some serious pain. It felt like breast pain in the days leading up to your period times about 10. There are things you can do to reduce the soreness though:

- Feed baby! – Even now at 3 months after delivery I get what is called let down pain – the milk comes down and I reach for Sumaya and latch her on for a feed. She's smiling content after a feed yet I find myself thanking her for the relief. If you don't plan on breastfeeding this will not be one of your chosen pain relief methods.

- Wearing a supportive bra

- Cabbage leaves in your bra – in the first few days these will add some extreme relief

- Shower/Bath

I do want to drum home though that breast feeding isn't supposed to hurt. I really recommend doing as much research about breastfeeding as a separate subject prior to labour.

We were readmitted into hospital with Sumaya not opening her bowels or urinating in the first 48 hours after birth. I was extremely scared thinking something was wrong but it was found to all be about her feeding, well my breastfeeding.

It turns out my colostrum wasn't actually feeding Sumaya enough. This was mainly due to how she was latching on. I was in excruciating pain feeding her but presumed it was what breastfeeding was supposed to feel like. Turns out she wasn't latching correctly and therefore not getting enough food which also was causing the pain. My nipples were extremely sore and if not bleeding were red raw. I would apply nipple cream and continue feeding.

The doctors involved in her care scanned her kidneys, intestines, liver and bowel looking for an obstruction. Turns out she just didn't have enough food in her system to cause her bowels or bladder to open. It was decided to give her formula as well as breast milk until my milk came through.

This knocked my confidence greatly and I was ready to hand the breastfeeding towel in. My milk finally arrived the same day that I was due to be discharged from the hospital. The midwife advised that I could stop using formula and instead express the same amount and feed Sumaya from a bottle.

I was really disappointed and wanted to breastfeed. I kept trying and getting frustrated would revert to the bottle. Just as I was packing up our bags to leave a lactation consultant arrived and asked if anyone needed her help.

I didn't know what a lactation consultant was but luckily one of the midwives mentioned I would be interested. It was honestly the best thing that could have happened.

The lactation consultant is a breastfeeding specialist. She watched how I was feeding first and then showed me step by step where I was going wrong and how I could fix the issues I was facing. Turns out my breasts are quite heavy so rather than hold Sumaya across my chest in the 'rock a by baby' position I'm better of holding her under my arm like a rugby ball.

It's amazing the difference it made. I not feel so comfortable, I can literally feed her anywhere. On the sofa, on the bed, in the car park, in Westfields shopping Centre; I have and continue to feed. No more grimaces or holding back the tears. It's a very comfortable rewarding process now.

Most hospitals will have one and if not will definitely be able to provide you with information on lactation consultants to assist if you choose to breastfeed. Even if you are a natural it's still worth having them check over your technique before you leave. You can always call the National Breastfeeding helpline for advice: 0300 100 0212

Baby Checks

Once Sumaya had been delivered (I didn't realize it) the midwifes performed a quick physical examination of her before she was put onto my chest for skin to skin contact.

They had done what is known as the APGAR score:

Appearance – Skin Colouration
Pulse- Heart Rate
Grimace – Irritability reflex
Activity – Muscle Tone
Respiration – Breathing rate and effort.

It is a simple check to assess how well the baby is doing. This is done straight after birth and then again at 5 and 10 minutes. It isn't designed to indicate any long term health issues but a quick assessment to decide if the baby needs any immediate treatment.

Each letter is given a score of between 1 and 2, with scores between 7 and 10 meaning baby doesn't require any treatment.

They then took her away to the other side of the room to weigh her, measure her height and measure her head circumference.

It was all done in the room with me and completely visible.

She was then given her Vitamin K shot.

Vitamin K

Vitamin K is used to ensure baby's blood clots properly. Newborns have less Vitamin K and without it are at risk of a bleeding disorder. The chance of this disorder is really low and as a result some parents decide not to give it to their baby.

This can be done as one injection or orally although if done orally it will need to be administered again. As mentioned you can opt for your baby not to have Vitamin K administered at all.

Before you are discharged from the hospital the baby will be checked by a doctor. They will check baby's eyes, hips, heart and physical appearance i.e. legs, arms and reflexes.

Newborn babies also have their hearing tested. This may not be done before you are discharged as you may be able to have it done as an outpatient. It is a painless procedure with small earphones put in baby's ear. The initial result is given straight away with any issues investigated.

In the days and weeks following the birth you will be visited by both a community midwifery team as well as a health visitor. This is either done at your home or at a local clinic.
It is an excellent opportunity to ask questions and raise any concerns.

Having a baby is a joyful experience with the beautiful end result of parenthood. No one said it was going to be easy though. I do hope I have helped you to feel able to deal with the coming months ahead leading up to the birth of your baby.

As an added bonus I have included a short summary of your baby's development from conception to delivery.

Baby Sizes week by week – real-world comparisons

Week	Size Comparison
4	Poppy Seed (2mm)
5	Sesame Seed (3mm)
6	Lentil (6mm)
7	Blueberry (1.2cm)
8	Kidney Bean (1.6cm) (1g)
9	Grape (2.3cm) (2g)
10	Green Olive (3.1cm) (4g)
11	Fig (4.1cm) (7g)
12	Lime (5.4cm) (14g)
13	Pea pod (7.4cm) (23g)
14	Lemon (8.7cm) (43g)
15	Apple (10.1cm) (70g)
16	Avocado (11.6cm) (100g)
17	Turnip (13cm) (140g)
18	Bell Pepper (14.2cm) (190g)
19	Heirloom Tomato (15.3cm) (240g)
20	Small Banana (25.6cm) (300g)
21	Carrot (26.7cm) (360g)
22	Squash (27.8cm) (430g)
23	Large Mango (28.9cm) (500g)
24	Ear of corn (30cm) (600g)
25	(34.6cm) Swede (660g)
26	(35.6cm) Red Cabbage (760g)
27	(36.6cm) Cauliflower (875g)
28	(37.6cm) Aubergine (1kg)
29	(38.6cm) Butternut Squash (1.2kg)
30	(39.9cm) Cabbage (1.3kg)
31	(41.1cm) Coconut (1.5kg)
32	(42.2cm) (1.7kg)
33	(43.7cm) Pineapple (1.9kg)
34	(45cm) Cantaloupe melon (2.1kg)
35	(46.2cm) Honeydew melon (2.4kg)
36	(47.4cm) (2.6kg)
37	(48.6cm) (2.9kg)
38	(49.8cm) (3kg+)

| 39 | (50.7cm) Watermelon (3.3kg) |
| 40 | (51.2cm) Pumpkin (3.5kg) |

*From about 20weeks the baby is measured from head to heel instead of crown to rump (head to bottom)

**From 25weeks we ran out of height comparisons and changed it to weight comparisons.

Development of your baby – From Conception to Delivery

Please note, this is a rough guide about what happens during the pregnancy. Baby's all develop differently. This is in no means a medical guide but a general idea of how development works.

Weeks 1 – 3

Although pregnancy is counted as the first day of your last period you won't have been pregnant during the first 3 weeks of pregnancy. Strange right? Around week three though the embryo implants into the lining of the womb. This is known as implantation and may result in a little bit of spotting sometimes known as implantation bleeding. This may be pink, or brown tinged. Some woman don't even notice it.

Week 4

The inner cells of the embryo form three layers. The inner layer becomes the breathing and digestive systems i.e. lungs, stomach. The middle layer becomes the heart, muscles and bones. The outer layer becomes the brain, nervous system, skin and nails.

At this stage the placenta hasn't formed yet. The embryo gains the nourishment from a tiny sac. The embryo is surrounded by fluid inside the amniotic sac. It's the outer layer of the sac that later becomes the placenta. The placenta will grow deep into the wall of the womb ensuring the developing baby receives oxygen and nutrients transferred from the mother.

Week 5

The baby's nervous system begins to develop now. The major organ's foundations are firmly in place even with the embryo only 2mm long. The beginnings of the baby's brain and spinal cord are also developing. Defects at the bottom end of this development can lead to Spina Bifida while defects at the top end can lead to the bones of the skull not forming properly.

The heart has also begun to form a simple version of its later self. With some of the blood vessels already developed the blood begins to circulate. A string of these blood vessels will later become the umbilical cord.

Week 6

At this stage your embryo begins to take on a tadpole like appearance. It has a large bulge where the heart is and a bump where the brain and head will end up being. It's at this stage a transvaginal ultrasound may be able to detect the heart beating.

Towards the end of this week little buds will being to appear. There will be swellings where the arms and legs will be as well as little dimples on the bud for the head. The little dimples indicate where the ears and eyes will be. The embryo will even have a layer of see through skin.

Week 7

By Week 7 the embryo is now around 10mm or 1cm. The brain is growing fastest and therefore the head is growing faster than the rest of the body. The head also has a large forehead as the eyes and ears continue to develop from week 6. Interestingly only the inner part of the ear has begun to develop so the outer parts of the ear don't yet appear.

Those limbs that were previous swellings begin to form cartilage which develops into the bones for the legs and arms. The arm buds are getting longer with the ends being flat to show where the hands will be.

Week 8

The embryo is now called a foetus meaning offspring. As the arms were getting longer last week, the legs now begin to get some length and forming cartilage. There isn't the separate parts of the legs yet it is one single shape.

The placenta has still not developed fully yet so the foetus is relying on the yolk sac for all its nourishment

Week 9

The face of the foetus is slowly beginning to come together. The eyes are larger and even have some pigment to them. There is a mouth and tongue. The tiny tongue even has even tinier taste buds.

The hands and feet which were previous flat shapes now have ridges to identify where the fingers and toes will be although they haven't actually separated yet. At 9 weeks the baby will average about 2.3cm or 23mm in length

Week 10

The outer part of the ear is beginning to develop on the outside of the head. On the inside of the head the ear canal is continuing to form.

Most importantly this week is the heart which is now fully formed. The heart is beating 2 to 3 times faster than your own heart at approximately 180 beats per minute.

The face also continues to develop. There will now be an upper lip and nostrils in the now forming nose. The milk teeth are already embedded deep into the developing jawbone.

Your baby is now making small movements which would be visible if you were to have an ultrasound scan.

Week 11

The foetus is continuing to develop with the placenta almost fully formed.

The bones that make your baby's face are now formed. The baby's head actually takes up a third of its length.

The body is growing rapidly in a bid to even things out though The hands and feet have now separated to show the fingers and toes. The fingers even have fingernails now.

Week 12

Ohhh week 12, is a particularly special one. The foetus is now fully formed. All the organs are in place as well as the muscles and limbs. Even the sex organs are developed although not fully.
The foetus is now a miniature version of the final baby, all that needs to happen is for all the parts to grow and mature.

The baby is moving around a lot even though it will be some time before you will be able to feel it.

The skeleton of the baby is still cartilage but will now being to develop into hard bone.

Week 13

The baby's reproductive organs are fully developed inside the body. The genitals are also forming outside of the body. There will be a swelling outside of the body which will later develop into the penis for a boy and clitoris for a girl. Even though these are developing it will be some weeks yet before you can scan to find out the gender of your baby.

Week 14

At around 14 weeks the baby will begin swallowing small amounts of the surrounding amniotic fluid. The kidneys have developed enough to begin passing this consumed amniotic fluid back out as urine. This will continue until the baby is born so it's not anything to worry about.

The facial muscles are continuing to develop and are being worked and experimented with. Your baby can frown, squint and even suck its thumb.

The thin layer of skin will start having the lanugo grow over his body. This is ultra-thin hair that will keep him warm inside the womb. The body is continuing to grow with the arms now in proportion with the rest of his body.

Week 15

Your baby will begin to hear, although it won't hear much from the outside world it will hear some. What your baby will hear is your digestive sounds and heartbeat. Your heartbeat will later provide a source of comfort after birth from the loud noises of the world.

It's not only the ears that begin to work, your baby's eyes will now become sensitive to light even though they remain closed. If you were to shine a light against your stomach the baby will likely move away from the source.

The legs now have grown longer than the arms and the baby will be able to move all of these limbs.

Week 16

Your baby's nervous system continues to develop, as the muscles and limbs are flexed and moved. Even your baby's hands can move now, and possibly even reach out and touch each other.

The eyes and ears are moving closer to their final position in the front and sides of the head.

A cute little note, the baby's toenails are now beginning to grow.

Week 17

Those sweat glands he'll come to hate as he grows into a teenager have now begun to develop all over his body.

A substance called myelin has begun wrapping around the spinal cord to protect it.

With the baby growing the umbilical cord becomes stronger and thicker connecting to the placenta to continue to transfer the oxygen and nutrients from mum to baby.

The rubbery cartilage of the skeletal structure continues to harden into bone.

The head and body are now more in proportion too.

Week 18

Baby's chest now moves up and down to mimic breathing. If you could see inside you'd see the baby's blood vessels visible through the skin.

Baby's reproductive organs are now developed and in place. If it's a girl, that means the vagina, fallopian and uterus and if it's a boy you'll be able to recognise his genitals on an ultrasound scan.

The ears are now also where they should be although they still stick out slightly. Their face looks more human like with eyebrows and eyelashes beginning to grow too. The eyes are moving, even though they are still closed. Even the mouth opens and closes.

Week 19

The hair on baby's scalp is now beginning to grow although it will be a while yet before you can see its colour and even that can change after birth.

The five senses are continuing to develop in the brain, that's taste, smell, hearing, seeing and touch. This reaches its peak this week as the more complex process develop at a slower rate.

The lines on the skin of the fingers are forming too. This means the baby already has its own individual fingerprints. As the fingernails grow so does the strength of the baby's grip.

<u>Week 20</u>

You may experience the fluttering movements of baby by now. This is known as quickening. What you may think is rumbling or wind may in fact be your baby moving around.

Don't worry if you haven't noticed the movements yet, first time mums don't always feel the movements as early as a woman that's been pregnant before.

At 20 weeks the skin begins to produce a protective coating called vernix. It is a white greasy substance that protects the skin sitting in all that fluid. You will notice it when the baby is born it's a nightmare to get out if the baby has hair.

<u>Week 21</u>

From now the baby will begin to put on weight although they will still have a wrinkled appearance. The weight of baby should now begin to be more than the placenta. Both will continue to grow but baby will just grow at a faster rate.

Baby will also begin taking in more amniotic fluid. This is to help train its digestive system. The water of the amniotic fluid will be taken out with the waste transferring to the bowel. It's this waste that will later make up the meconium passed after birth.

In terms of movement you may begin to notice a pattern to baby's movement. This is unlikely to follow your pattern of day and night. In most cases it will actually be the opposite with the majority of baby's movement occurring when you're resting or even trying to sleep.

Week 22

Baby finally looks like a new born with all the parts in the right place although not all are fully developed – specifically the lungs.

This doesn't stop baby from practising his breathing technique in preparation for life outside of the womb. Don't worry though, the placenta is still providing all the oxygen baby needs

Baby mainly needs to put on weight from now until birth. Baby's skin is still very wrinkled although the curled up position is beginning to straighten out.

Facially the baby has distinct lips and eyes, with the eyes just needing their pigment to develop. They are still closed though.

Week 23

Baby can now recognise your voice. You could try singing or talking to your bump. It may feel a little strange initially but you'll soon get used to it. Loud noises such as the hoover or dog barking will be normal for the baby when they are born if they are used to hearing them inside the womb. They will remember and recognise the sounds.

The lungs are continuing to develop and the baby is continuing to get bigger (you can refer to my size table). Some women are even able to see baby's movements underneath their clothes!

Week 24

By now the baby has a chance of survival if they were born around now. They will require a lot of assistance and have to stay in hospital for a long time but the chance of survival is definitely there.

As medicine advances are made the care available in the neonatal units is too, meaning more babies are surviving.

Baby's brain and lungs continue to develop with the lungs developing the cells needed to inflate the air sacs after birth.

Week 25

From around 25 weeks you may begin to notice the baby jumping or kicking in response to loud noises. Sometimes baby's also get hiccups which can feel a bit like a bubbling sensation. If so you will be able to feel every single hiccup – it is both very strange and quite comical. Don't worry though it's not hurting them.

Baby will also begin putting on weight and start exchanging the wrinkled look for a more lean appearance.

Week 26

Baby will now be very interested in hearing you speak and may begin to remember other voices too of those they hear often i.e. a partner or parent. The response to sound and light continues to develop and become more sophisticated as the brain develops.

At around the 26th week your baby may open its eyes. They will soon begin practising blinking. In terms of the eye colour they may not have their permanent eye colour yet with most babies being born with blue or dark blue eyes.

Week 27

Baby now should have a regular sleeping pattern. Your baby may also begin sucking its thumb. At around now I had a scan which showed Sumaya sucking her toes.

Baby is now also an expert at opening and closing their eyes.

Although faster than yours the baby's heartbeat begins to slow down around now to approximately 140bpm

Week 28

Baby now has eyelashes. Their bones are nearly fully developed although they are not exactly hard. They will harden after baby is born

Baby is regularly turning her head in the womb usually away from the light of outside.

The important fat layers are continuing to develop although baby is not at its final birth weight yet.

Week 29

At this stage the baby's head begins to get bigger as the brain grows in size also.

The sexual organs continue to grow also with the boy's testicles moving down into place through the groin. For a girl the clitoris appears larger as the outer labia is still quite small. This will be in proportion during the last few weeks before birth.

Week 30

The lanugo which kept your baby at the right temperature begins to disappear in preparation for the birth. The white greasy substance also begins to disappear although traces will still be visible after birth.

At this stage the movements of baby will be very active as they should still have some space to kick around. The amniotic fluid lessens as the baby grows in size. There is only so much room in the uterus.

Baby continues to open and close its eyes although they can only see small distances ahead. They have probably seen all of what's going on inside of your uterus though.

The digestive tract is now almost fully developed

Week 31

Baby's lungs are developing at a rapid rate although they won't be fully developed for a few weeks yet.

Baby's movements may begin to slow down around now as the space in the womb begins to run out. You should still feel wriggling and kicking though.

Baby will also be weeing regularly now

Week 32

From around 32 weeks the chance of survival is quite high, with the chance of baby being born with a disability decreasing.

Baby's lungs are beginning to practise the art of breathing by taking in amniotic fluid.

By the end of the 32 week most babies have their head down in preparation for birth. If not there is still time and your midwife will check at appointments to make sure it's the case.

The hair on babies head is now also prominent. Some babies are born with loads, others with little or none. All are quite normal.

Week 33

Baby's brain is now fully developed. The baby may also begin to move head down into your pelvis.

The skeletal structure is also continuing to harden with the skull still soft to allow for the journey through the birth canal. The skull bones will be able to glide over one another while still protecting the brain to allow for safe delivery.

Week 34

Baby is getting rounder with their fat layer building up. This will help regulate their body temperature when born. They will now also have soft and smoother skin having filled out the wrinkled appearance.

Week 35

Baby's hearing is now fully developed. They also have fully grown finger and toenails. The liver is actively working to process the waste products.
With space now minimised you may notice an elbow or foot protruding from your belly as your little one squirms and stretches.

Week 36

The lungs are finally fully developed. They are fully formed and ready to begin working outside of the womb.
The digestive system is also prepared to deal with the first feed of breast milk with baby able to suckle for feeds around now too.

Week 37

Pregnancies are considered full term from around now. Your baby's head is now in your pelvic area. The baby has digested the lanugo and vernix which will make up the meconium found in the first nappy. This is currently being stored in the baby's bowels.

Week 38

Baby continues to put on weight building up their fat stores. Their lungs are still practising in anticipation for the impending birth.

Week 39

The wait continues, baby is still shedding the vernix turning the amniotic fluid from clear to a milky colour. Baby's skin is coming off as new skin forms underneath.

Baby's genital area may appear swollen, this is just down to hormones and will soon sort itself out after birth. It's not anything to worry about.

Week 40

Baby may still be in the womb waiting to be born. It's pretty comfortable in there, it's warm and snug. They will continue to grow and put on weight and relax probably. Especially if it's your first baby anyway.

If baby is a little late they may be born with dry skin as most of the vernix will have gone by then. I personally recommend olive oil as this cleared up Sumaya's skin in no time. When first suggested by a midwife I couldn't believe it, actual olive oil, like what you dress salad with and cook with? Yes, it really works.

Printed in Great Britain
by Amazon.co.uk, Ltd.,
Marston Gate.